"Having served on the front li[ne]... life, I can say that *Dare to be K...* ...tion of a gritty true life story of honesty, perseverance and resilience that will resonate with so many. Although Melanie could have surrendered many times, she chose to not be a victim or casualty but a true warrior at heart. After reading this book, the raw emotions Melanie shared will impact the way you think, interpret and respond to life's critical challenges."

—Al Gray - *RCMP (Retired), Vancouver, B.C.*

"As a mental health practitioner, I gained so much insight into the struggles that my patients must go through and I feel like your story will definitely make me a better nurse. Thank you for putting yourself out there so that others may benefit from your experiences."

—Sandra MacCuaig - *Mental Health and Addictions Nurse, Cornwall, ON*

"An unflinchingly honest, gutsy and compelling true life story! A must read!"

—Maxwell McGuire - *Writer & Film Director, Ottawa, ON*

"This book gave me tremendous insight on issues that teens face. I feel better equipped with applicable strategies to know how to support my kids through this confusing and difficult stage of life. A must read for all parents who feel helpless and don't know what to do. This book gave me reassurance, peace and hope that we aren't the only ones struggling and that we too can and will make it through this season."

—Mother - *of a teen struggling with low self-esteem, self-injury and depression, Ottawa, ON*

"Thank you for being unusually honest, human and brave. This book is so much more than just a memoir, but will serve as a rich tool for many caregivers out there!"

—Rachelle Gagnon - *Registered Nurse, Royal Alexandra Hospital Emergency, Edmonton, AB*

"A brave depiction of the debilitating impact of trauma and the hope that we can *fully* recover from it. One to never abandon hope, Melanie Willard has just contributed wisdom, beauty and life to the human race."

—Dustin Nau - *Ph.D Psychology, Calgary, AB*

"One of the sad global realities is that so many long for a 'second chance' in life that will deliver hope and contentment. Melanie Willard is a true champion in heart, soul and mind...a woman of integrity and courage who has overcome the unthinkable. What an encouragement her testimony will be to those privileged to read *Dare to be Raw*. She has been an inspiration to me as we have shared 'war' stories over coffee. God is the One who delivers our 'second chances'. "

—Gerry Organ - *Former CFL Athlete, Therapist, Pastor and Author, Ottawa, ON*

"Melanie's raw account of her life's journey is a true portrayal of courage and compassion. She speaks her truth for us the readers to transform our own reality into opportunities for growth and change. This book will leave you empowered!"

—Katherine MacDonald - *Owner & Grief Care Provider at Munro Morris Funeral Home, Alexandria, ON*

"Melanie's journey speaks of the seemingly impossible becoming possible. Thanks to her transparency, this very human story is one that we can all identify with on some level. This book causes us to reflect and look in the mirror of our own lives while building the fortitude to embrace our pain and move from despair to hope. A truly inspiring and moving read that will impact many."

—Danell Mcsween - *Founder and Consultant at OIL-Operating In Love, Calgary, AB*

Melanie's heartbreaking story is filled with glimpses of hope interrupted by deep grief. Her courageous honesty is inspirational, encouraging each of us to accept ourselves in our humanness. Melanie's authentic rawness offers insight and support to others on a similar quest for healing. Thank you, Melanie, for Daring to be Raw and giving us this opportunity to draw inspiration and hope for ourselves from your journey.

Michelle Bentley, MA
Registered Marriage & Family Therapist, Ottawa, ON

DARE TO BE RAW

DARE TO BE RAW

A True Story of Triumph Over Tragedy

Growing in resilience and hope while journeying
through the battlefields of life.

♡melanie willard

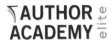

I dedicate this book to you the reader.
Wherever you are in your journey I encourage you to be yourself,
never give up hope and know you are loved beyond measure.

CONTENTS

FOREWORD

We all long for love and acceptance.

So many of us screech at the thought of expressing and being our true authentic selves. We wear masks as we strive for perfection and people pleasing at all costs. We silence our urge to scream that "Everything is NOT OK!" As a result we communicate through silent coping mechanisms. Unfortunately the result has been painful for many and it almost cost Melanie Willard, her life.

I believe our deepest wounds are often the place where we'll have the deepest impact upon others. Our pain doesn't disqualify us. It makes us credible and believable.

That said, one could award author Melanie Willard with a PhD in the school of hard knocks.

Melanie is a walking testimony of what it means to be resilient and to truly bounce back from not one crisis, but multiple life threatening and destiny altering events.

Melanie's candid and honest story has a way of tearing down the walls built around our hearts. As you read you will likely look back at your own life and how you dealt and coped with your own losses. Melanie shares nuggets of wisdom she has earned and learned along the way that will help you improve future responses.

You will gain greater understanding of the snowball effect that one bad decision can have upon your life. And you will understand the healing and redemptive roles that honesty and vulnerability play in all human interactions.

Melanie has laid her soul bare. She is daring us to do the same and as a result experience restored relationships, deepened intimacy, renewed joy, untamable freedom, and unshakable peace. She challenges us to get out from under the shame of our bondage and silent addictions and live in the light and freedom that results from being honest with ourselves and the world around us.

Melanie is a brave warrior whose battle cry is to always tell the truth, to always be yourself, and to never give up hope no matter what.

Kary Oberbrunner
Author of *ELIXIR Project*, *Day Job to Dream Job*, *The Deeper Path*, and *Your Secret Name*

INTRODUCTION

"I now see how owning our story and loving ourselves
through that process is the bravest thing
that we will ever do."
—Brené Brown

For the title of this book to have any meaning or value, I cannot shy away from being true to my story, sharing the good, the bad, and the ugly. I cannot take the safe path but rather the road less travelled, by laying my life bare. Through my transparency, I hope you will give yourself permission to embrace your own humanness, as we celebrate both the fragility and resilience of the human spirit. I must refrain from deleting any of the passages I fear may be uncomfortable, unpleasant, offensive, or even unbelievable to you.

I sit here in my chair with my computer on my lap, having just spoken with a friend who gave me feedback on my first chapter. Basically, she said my book was anything but *raw*. Just what I wanted to hear! Apparently, it was much too calculated, as though I was sharing intellectually rather than from my heart. A part of me is yelling loudly in protest of exposing and baring my soul to a world that can be such a mean and nasty place. The risk and fear of judgment or rejection is an overwhelming one for me.

So, here goes take two! This time with a lump in my throat, my insides shaking, and tears welling up. Yes, I'm afraid and petrified of what could come out of this. I second guess myself as I think, "Why am I putting myself through this?" It's my sincere desire that the potential backlash of writing this book will be faint in comparison to the impact it will have on you. If you find hope and courage to continue on your journey, then this gnawing discomfort will have been worth it to me. I trust you will glean wisdom and tools from my life lessons, learning "what not to do" and how to avoid pitfalls in your own life.

As I sit here and look back at how far I have come, my heart is overwhelmed with gratitude. The fact that I am still here to share my story with you is nothing short of a miracle.

CHAPTER 1

All the Ingredients for a Happy Life; What went wrong?

"Why are you in despair, O my soul? And why
have you become disturbed within me?"
—Psalm 42:5

First off, everything in this book is 100% true. And although it is an honest account of trials, tragedy, and suffering, it is equally full of triumph, adventure, and beauty. So stick with me through the tough parts, because it all turns around for the best! I promise! We will walk through some deep waters together, but only to soar like eagles in the end.

In case you start to question my sanity at any point in this book, I am your average girl next door. I have no mental illness, and never suffered abuse or trauma when I was younger. It is crucial for me to start from the beginning for you to understand the hardships and trials I have endured. While some were self-inflicted, others were completely out of my control.

I grew up in a French Canadian home in very small town between Montreal and Ottawa. We used to joke that if you blinked while passing through, you would miss it!

Growing up, our home was full of life, love, and peace. We were an ordinary and traditional family with no fireworks to report. I grew up with all the ingredients for a happy life! So what went wrong?

Why was I so sad and violently restless within?
Where did this inner discontent and torment come from?

My parents owned a successful reception hall for nine years while Dad also taught music at the local high school. He was a respected entrepreneur as well as a very effective teacher and gifted musician. Dad was a strong leader, hard-working, affectionate, and loving. He gave me all the traits I didn't want, like his hypersensitivity, his "griz-like" body hair, and muscular legs.

Mom, on the other hand, was not the emotional type, as I could probably count the number of times I have seen her cry. A nurse by profession, Mom was a true nurturer, positive, generous, and loving. She wanted to live out her dream of becoming a figure skater through me but I, on the other hand, wanted nothing to do with it. She was left with a reckless, sport- and dirt-loving tomboy who rode her three-wheeler on her brother's motocross track.

My brothers were five and six years older which was enough of an age gap to mean I was on my own a lot. The oldest was the intellectual, a musical genius, and a natural athlete. He was the introverted, mysterious and closed off type. Today he is a musician, conductor, and professor in Georgia. Meanwhile, the younger brother was the driven extrovert who was the life of the party and had more friends than I had hair on my head. Today, he is an ambitious and very successful entrepreneur with a big and generous heart.

Regardless of the motley crew we grow up with, every family has its quirks, strengths and weaknesses. Since we were well known in our community, I struggled to be myself and found it impossible to come out from under the shadow of my family's identity and reputation. Instead, I fought hard to be what I thought everyone wanted me to be.

My parents were both high achieving perfectionists. They had high standards for themselves and their roles, and even though it was never directly imposed upon me, I came under those expectations. I remember striving for perfection but also striving for their love and acceptance. I had a very unhealthy fear of disappointing and displeasing my parents. I felt I had to be the perfect child and because of that I never rebelled or acted out like normal teenagers do.

My true self was dying inside, and I had a deep sense of emptiness like a dark hole that could not be filled. Being an imposter was absolutely exhausting, and the more I pretended to be happy the harder it was to stop playing the game. It takes a brave soul to embrace and expose its true nature. Vulnerability is one of the most freeing and underestimated qualities we can possess.

To say I was a highly sensitive child would be an understatement, and it served me as both a blessing and a curse. Although my tomboy exterior fought hard to protect its tough image, I used to weep as I watched the musical "Annie" or the movie "Benji" at school. I remember one girl who did cry and was bullied for it. So right away, I concluded that it wasn't safe for me to be myself.

Perhaps being tender-hearted was a quality, but at the time it was a total inconvenience and pain in the arse. I fought so hard to keep my composure, but inside me was an uncontrollable volcano of tears wanting to erupt.

Why was I so different?
Why couldn't I be normal like everybody else?

Not giving myself permission to voice my true feelings and "be myself" caused me to self-express in very destructive ways down the road.

If you are struggling with being or expressing yourself today, take my advice and *stop* right now! You have no choice but to be brave enough to be the real *you*. If people can't accept and love you for the way you are, then they don't deserve to take up space in your world. Life is too short to live any other way than as your authentic and unique self.

Tender Heart

One hot summer morning, I remember walking through the parking lot of our reception hall/home. I came across a dying little bird who was suffering and struggling for every breath. I went to get some water, and when I got back, it was dead. You can imagine what happened next. I cried as if I had known that bird as a pet for years! Pathetic, I know, but it is true. I figured it deserved as much dignity as any of us, so I conducted my own funeral service. Out came the shovel as I wept and dug a hole, and wept some more until, finally, I laid it down to rest. Then I asked God to be reunited with it in Heaven one day.

On other occasions, I would channel surf, and my heart would get ripped out of my chest from watching starving children on World Vision commercials. This sense of guilt and sorrow would flood over me to the point where I couldn't even watch them and still can't to this day! I felt as though life was handed to me on a silver platter while so many people were fighting for their lives daily. How could I possibly enjoy life knowing there were so many people suffering in this world? These toxic thoughts led me to become a burden-bearer thinking that maybe if I suffered, perhaps my pain could help alleviate theirs. It was a warped saviour mentality that ended up almost costing me my life. Remember, this is coming from a five-year-old kid.

Christmas was a dreaded holiday for me. The small flickers of joy were overshadowed by an overwhelming sense of guilt and sadness as I thought about the kids who weren't so lucky. Opening presents felt awkward and uncomfortable. I wished I could give Santa a piece of my mind. "Like, come on, Dude—why are you so generous with some and not with others?" It felt unjust. I remember going up to my room once the festivities were over feeling so deflated, sad, confused, and helpless. Again, all the ingredients for a normal and happy childhood gone bad, and it was nobody's fault.

Brave Heart

Another dominant trait of mine was my insatiable need for adventure! I had (and still have) a deep desire to be part of a bigger story, to save the day, to kill the bad guys, and to somehow make a difference in this world. I would climb trees and build forts; for me to play with dolls and makeup was not appealing but appalling! The more branches, dirt, and rocks involved in my playtime the better!

The imaginary scenarios I entertained in my mind came to life through my Barbie dolls. They co-starred with Sylvester Stallone in *First Blood* as they fought the bad guys and were rescued by their heartthrob and fearless warrior, John Rambo. These Barbies never went to the spa—they got dirty, scraped, and bruised during their fight for survival in my backyard and were officially baptised "Rambettes."

Can you hear the Indiana Jones and Rocky soundtracks playing in the background? I was an adventure, adrenaline, and extreme sports junky. Although that part of me is still alive and kicking today, I'm learning to restrain myself now that I have a family. Plus, I refuse to have to recover from yet another injury.

Unusual Encounters

Much of what I've been through is abnormal, complex, and even supernatural in nature. My challenge as I write is to articulate or paint an accurate picture of my experiences without confusing you too much or coming across like a total freak. Since God has been such a big part of my life, it's impossible for me to leave Him out to appease everyone. That would be like leaving myself out of my own story. I just can't do it.

I wasn't much of an artist growing up, but I do remember the one thing I did draw. Faces. Not just any faces, but the images of spirits that I saw. Dark, gothic, monster-looking beings like creepy goblins out of a horror movie. Don't ask me why or where it came from! It is still a mystery to me today.

I remember one event in particular that was perhaps the onset of many wounds to come. Growing up, I had a serious dislike for anything to do with the 70s decade and culture. The drugs, the colours, the music all left me feeling dirty.

I was around five or six years of age, and we were at a party in a dark basement. It was a typical 70s party with the disco music blasting, the loud carpet and outfits, and a room full of normal people drinking and dancing the night away. Nothing abnormal or evil.

However, I remember feeling alone, disconnected from what was happening in the room like I was watching a movie. The music became a blur, and I was just standing there when all of a sudden my spiritual eyes were opened, and I saw not the pretty faces dancing, but demons or skeletal structures surface within the faces. They were what I can only describe as lustful, seducing spirits.

You are probably thinking, "What the heck?!" I know it's weird, but seriously, why in my right mind would I ever make this up? I wish this weren't part of my story, but to understand future events, this story helps set the stage. The irony of it all is that I have never shared this with anyone before except for one counsellor out of fear of being dismissed, rejected, or mocked. And here I am today reluctantly sharing it with the world.

If you've seen the movie *The Devil's Advocate* with Keanu Reeves and Al Pacino, then you may recall a couple of scenes where they showed the demonic spirits revealed through the natural and pretty faces of women. When I saw it 20 years ago, I wondered where the director got that idea. Perhaps through his own experience? I found it interesting that how I saw spirits (and still see, at times) was perfectly depicted in that movie. Now, I am not endorsing or recommending this film, by any means! It is dark, and no walk in the park, so be forewarned.

Should you ever feel lured and tempted by the beautiful outer shell of a person, more than just normal attraction, *perhaps* it is a spirit trying to seduce you. Do yourself a favor and look past the surface, as it is likely on a mission sent to tempt you and to destroy your life. I am not saying it is the case every time, but it can happen!

Let's go back to the disco party for a moment. I wasn't afraid or wigged out or anything. To me, it was as natural as the clothes we wear. It was the feeling associated with the view that disturbed me. Although I was never raped physically as a child, this experience marked me, stained me, and left me owning the same feelings as though I had been violated. I felt defiled, dirtied, and slimed by the situation as if their lust was transferred to me.

This played a significant role in the eating disorders I developed later on in my teens. After much fruitless therapy, one day in my late twenties I was at a prayer/counselling session and the veil was lifted. I understood what had happened. I saw a vision through prayer of Jesus with me in the disco room. I had believed that the spirits had defiled and entered my being, but that was not the truth. It was as if I revisited that place in prayer, and this time, even though the spirits were there, they had no power over me. I saw myself as a white lamb, clean, pure, and untainted. The filth was no longer allowed to touch me, and this little girl was cleansed and restored. That truth set me free.

Have you ever been in love with someone? To compartmentalise the emotions and feelings attached to love and translate them into words is hard, isn't it? It almost feels like it reduces its full value, true nature, and beauty right? It was only after I fell in love that I could understand what it felt like to be IN love. Same with the spiritual. It's not a cerebral experience that can be properly described. We as human beings can be so quick to judge what we don't comprehend because of our lack of experience.

I'll do my best to describe some of these stories, but if you don't understand, that's OK. Just come along for the ride, and I guarantee you will be inspired in the end.

It was after this disco party experience that my senses were awakened more consistently to the unseen realms. My desire to hide my body became more extreme. I *know* for a fact that many women have experienced what I am about to share. Some individuals have lustful or perverted spirits within them. Have you ever felt someone undress you with their eyes, or look right through your clothes?

When that would happen to me, I would curse under my tongue. To prevent them from raping me with their eyes, I started hiding under baggy clothes, even Dad's clothes, but it didn't seem to help. This fueled my anger like nothing else. I would feel dirty, slimed, defiled, shamed, and just plain *yuck*.

For years, I did not know how to handle that. I would look at them with laser eyes like the Terminator repelling them as best as I could. I felt helpless to the point where I even told a couple of guys to F-off. Thankfully what has worked for me over the last decade is a simple prayer, and Jesus is faithful to cleanse me every time. He is awesome like that.

At this point, my distorted image and tough tomboy persona were setting deep roots in me. I felt I had to maintain it to avoid any form of mockery. Any hope or desire to wear makeup or feminine clothes became a pipe dream. Deep inside it felt so unfair, as though I had been robbed of my femininity. I did not wish to be a boy, but I wasn't too happy about being a girl either.

In all honesty, what I wanted was to become *invisible.*

Why was everyone else free to be normal girly girls, while I was too insecure and scared of people's reaction if I stepped out of my tomboy image? I fed this false identity and felt more and more anger towards others and myself for not being free to be me. This bottled up anger soon turned to rage, and that rage turned against itself and gave birth to various self-destructive behaviors.

The Green Giant

As a little girl, I was everything *but* little. I felt like the green giant, as I was taller than the majority of my classmates, which just fed my already wounded and negative self-image. I was just not a "cute" kid and don't remember ever feeling pretty. I was far from petite or delicate. To say I loathed every ounce of my being is an understatement.

Even though I was a popular and normal girl with a healthy social life, inside I *felt* like an outsider and a misfit.

I'm sure I wasn't the only one who felt flawed, awkward and ugly but of course I wasn't going to make it a public announcement. The result was that I felt all alone in my struggle, and thought everyone else loved who they were. I envied the pretty girls, compared myself to their smaller frames and wished I could be just like them. I figured if I looked like them I would be happier.

To be honest, I haven't grown an inch since I was twelve. I was only nine when "congratulations," I was officially a woman! Just what I wanted: my period, B.O., a growing bosom, and feeling different and alone in my development yet again. It wasn't until years later, when the rest of the girls began to develop, that I could let the cat out of the bag and bring the secrecy of my womanhood to an end. Most girls in elementary school had "boyfriends" but I felt like one of the boys. So the fact that I was never "pursued" reinforced that I was flawed. In my mind, I wasn't "purdy" and I felt like an undesirable butch.

Loss and hardships are unavoidable in life, however, "how" we deal with our pain is what will make us or break us. When wounded, we either become casualties of life or we learn to embrace and overcome our aches with dignity and triumph. On a mission to self-destruct most of my days, I have finally made peace with myself and seek to inspire you to do the same. Our lives are a perfect depiction of the pendulum between both the fragility and resilience of the human spirit. I hope my story will spark some grit and a fresh hope in you to never give up, no matter what!

I have been at peace with myself and at war with myself. Peace is better.

> "Don't bury the treasure of your life under the opinions and expectations of strangers."
> —Lisa Bevere

CHAPTER 2

Masked: The Cost of Being an Imposter

"The privilege of a lifetime is to
become who you truly are."
—C.G. Jung

If I could talk to my old teen self, I would sit her down, look her right in the eyes, remove her mask, and set her free from her self-imposed prison. Be brave, girl, and be yourself! Life is difficult enough fulfilling our own role, let alone trying to fill someone else's shoes.

Somehow, deep down I felt that if people saw my raw colours, they would be appalled. I believed I was flawed, and in order to please everyone I always had to be "happy," behave perfectly, and never say no. My true identity had to remain hidden because surely it would be unacceptable.

I was confused.

Wasn't life good? I had nothing to complain about! Why was I so sad and hurting inside when the world around me was full of love and blessings? It didn't make sense to me. And I concluded that if I didn't understand the source of my own pain, how could I expect anyone else to make sense of it? As a result, I never gave my suffering a voice. Unfortunately, it found its own years later.

Students get diplomas when they graduate from high school, but I think they should also get diplomas for simply surviving the teen years. With all the hormones flying around and the constant pressure to perform and fit in, no wonder so many teens are confused, hurting, and self-medicating. Growing up in a good home doesn't make you immune to depression or other struggles. I have less concern for the teen who rebels, has tantrums, and expresses himself than the people pleaser who pretends like everything is OK but in reality is dying inside.

The Imposter Led Me into a Major Depression

If you surveyed my high school classmates, I am pretty sure none of them would have guessed that I was depressed and suicidal in high school. On the contrary, I had lots of friends, was highly involved in music and sports, and worked on weekends. I was a perfectionist and high achiever with a self-imposed need to be the perfect child, student, worker, and athlete.

To make mistakes or disappoint was never an option. Perfection was an impossible and exhausting goal to achieve and maintain. I probably had slight chemical imbalances in my growing brain like many other teens, as I remember being on top of the world one minute and wanting to end my life the next.

I know I had enough testosterone to go head-to-head with a bull, and my PMS days were monthly visits from hell. My late husband said it was a like a switch that would turn on and off. When it was over, he said it was as though that dark cloud had lifted, and his wife would return to him.

After years of not being or expressing myself, my depression grew worse by the day. I was so pent up, I had anger boiling on the inside and the only way I could let it out was by beating myself up. While every other kid was acting out, I was turning my emotions against myself. Remember, I was highly sensitive, and just the thought of displeasing or letting anyone down was enough for me to wear that mask at all costs. God forbid my humanness, imperfections, and weaknesses be exposed!

My main group of friends were the normal crowd. Parties, boyfriends—just living the typical teenage life. I never felt like I fit in. My heart was longing for something more, something this world maybe couldn't offer.

C.S. Lewis put words in my mouth when he said, "I have found a desire within myself that no experience in this world can satisfy; the most probable explanation is that I was made for another world."

In high school, I was fortunate enough to make three new friends. For the first time in my life, I was able to expose the real me and was fully embraced for who I was. It was refreshing, to say the least. They seemed to "get" me, and I got them. They had the ability to be goofy normal teenage girls, and on the flip side, they had a depth about them that allowed us to have some pretty deep and meaningful conversations that were very fulfilling.

Self-hatred and the Onset of a Life-Threatening Eating Disorder

By grade 11, I was really uncomfortable in my own skin. I felt as though I couldn't attract the guys I thought I liked, but the second a guy showed any interest in me, I would push him away because I could not receive love. You've probably heard the saying, "You can't love others until you love yourself." Well, I say you *can* love others if you don't love yourself. But I believe you will be incapable of *receiving* love until you love yourself.

I went on the occasional date and had two short-term relationships. But deep down I knew they weren't marriage material, so I just didn't see the point of dating for the sake of dating. I felt as though I had better things to do than waste their time and mine.

I still felt like the green giant and a big blob, even though most of my friends were now the same height or taller than I was. The anger from my lack of self-expression was all consuming, and my mission to self-destruct really took off.

Banging your head against a wall wasn't just an expression for me, it was a reality. When I found myself alone, I would literally bang my head against the wall, pull my hair out, and cry from the innermost depths of my being. I felt trapped, like a prisoner in my own body. I was revolting against who I was and what I looked like. The thoughts of self-hatred and lies were deafening. Nothing audible, of course, but it was like a nonstop tape playing in my head. The anger soon turned to unbearable rage within.

Being fake was an exhausting role to play and infuriating one to maintain.

I remember having an appetite inside of me that could not be filled or satisfied. I always had this sense that there was no bottom to my stomach. Even in high school, I remember thinking this deep hole in my stomach could only be filled by something from another world, because whatever food I ingested never filled or satisfied. I felt like I could have eaten nonstop to fill that empty hole in me.

My distorted body image started to be a problem. Slowly, I began calculating everything I was putting in my mouth. If I couldn't be in control of my own "raw" self, then at least I could control my food intake. We all know that lack of nutrition affects our brain function and health; my depression started to escalate. By the time I was in grade 12, I was in rough shape, but my "imposter" did not let on that anything was wrong. The fraud within did its job all too well.

The more I became obsessed with my body and all its flaws, the more I isolated myself. My friends would go out to the bars, and the majority of the time I opted to stay home. I would either watch horror movies by myself or lock myself in my room and workout for hours.

The more I isolated myself, the more I wanted to be alone.

Worlds at War—A Strange Infatuation with Death

A major component in my life that I have yet to mention is my spiritual appetite. As far back as I can remember I always had faith, and church was a place of refuge for me. I never doubted for a day that God existed. However, the church we attended was more about the "dos and don'ts," and I guess you could say I never really encountered God. But trust me, it wasn't for my lack of trying!

> "Our desire becomes insatiable because we have taken our longing for the Infinite and placed it upon finite things."
> —John Eldredge

We occasionally had confession at school, and if I happened to forget to do my prayers of penance, I honestly thought I was going to hell. As if my works would qualify or disqualify me from being acceptable to God! It was a bunch of crap, but I was bound to those beliefs and fuelled by those fears as if God's love for me was dependant on me being His perfect child. Sound familiar? Apparently, my fears concerning God were quite similar to fears about my earthly parents. I concluded that I was only pleasing and lovable as long as I was happy and behaving perfectly.

To me, life was much more than just the physical realm or what was visible to the natural eye. I always believed there had to be a creator because this world was far too complex, intricately sustained, and breathtaking to have just been an accident. Even though I didn't always "see" the other realm as vividly as I did in the disco room, my senses were very keen. The majority of the time it was like I could *feel, smell* and *see* the presence of good and evil, like a knowing or awareness.

And since my pursuit of God never amounted to anything, I figured I would explore and hopefully find Him through other means. I'd say to myself, "If You are truly the God of the universe, the creator of heaven and earth, surely You can talk to me and touch me! Let me hear, see, touch, and feel You! If You are who You say You are, and nothing is impossible for You, then why wouldn't You communicate with me, Your daughter."

It felt like my prayers or conversations with God were a one-way street. It was as though my words would hit the ceiling and never reach Him because I never got a response back. I couldn't hear His voice, and I never felt His presence or touch.

Can you imagine having that kind of relationship with your wife or husband?

Eventually, you would get frustrated and seek elsewhere for that relationship and intimacy! I was never taught in church that this type of relationship with God was even possible. Nobody I knew had that relationship with Him, so there was no proof that it was even an attainable goal. I was hungry for God, and I believe He put that desire in me in the first place. Actually, I believe we all have it, some of us just choose to ignore it more than others. I felt as though He was playing hide and seek with me, and I just couldn't seem to find Him.

Being a tenacious bulldog, that didn't stop me.

In my anger and frustration, I began seeking Him through the occult: spirit guides, Ouija boards, and psychics. I became obsessed with the "other" world, wanting to get as close to death as possible and live to tell about it. I figured if I couldn't find God in this realm, I would go find Him in His!

The line from the film *Flatliners* was my motto: "Today is a good day to die." The movie was about medical students who "died" for a few minutes and brought one another back to life to tell about their experience. I got it. I wanted it. I was on the same mission, except my story wasn't a movie.

I spent time in abandoned homes, churches, and cemeteries. I was desperate to connect with the other world, and went anywhere that I thought would provide easy access to it.

I had a few out-of-body experiences, which you are the first to hear about along with the rest of the world. One night, lying in bed, I remember my spirit being lifted to the ceiling of my room while my body lay below. I wasn't scared or anything, but nothing else happened, which was more of a concern for me. What was the point of that? This event took place a couple of times, and it all seemed very pointless. One time, my spirit even went outside of the house, which was a bit more intense as I could see my body lying in my bed through the house walls. I thought, "Ok, where is this going?" Again, nothing happened, at least that I was aware of.

In grade 11, I was driving back from a friend's place around midnight. I was near my home, but (as embarrassed as I am, I need to admit) I was lost and confused. I was alone, and somehow I ended up on a logging road with bush on both sides. There were no houses in what appeared to be the middle of nowhere. At this point, I was wondering where I was and how I even got there! And no I was not drunk.

I am not kidding you when I say this, but there was a wrestling match going on in the car. I was no longer alone. I felt the presence of "others," what I believe was good and evil, angels and demons, going hard at it. It was like two worlds at war, right in front of me. I knew it was serious when the car started driving itself, and the breaks no longer worked no matter how hard I pumped them.

I couldn't keep my hands on the steering wheel as it moved back and forth violently. It felt completely out of control. I felt my back held against the seat, and I could no longer move. I was a little wigged out at this point as I watched this gong show take place in front of me. I remember thinking to myself, "I am a healthy, normal human being, and this is really happening!"

It felt as though it was a fight to take me out. Although I didn't speak out loud, I remember thinking, "Jesus." I didn't want to get in the middle of this spiritual altercation, so I just let it run its course. Finally, the rollercoaster ride came to an end and almost immediately everything calmed down. I had control of the wheel once again, and the breaks finally worked. I stopped the car and wept—scared, shaking, confused, and probably still in shock. I ended up finding my way home and never told a soul about this little episode.

Depression's Deepest and Final Pit: Suicide

"I am worn out from sobbing. All night I flood my bed
with weeping, drenching it with my tears."
—Psalm 6:6 NLT

That was me. I sobbed in bed the majority of nights, and I still don't know why to this day. I remember weeping, with groans that can't be put into words and yet with no clue as to why. It was a debilitating and profound sadness that seemed to flood over me, inside, and around me. I could not escape its grip, its influence, or its gnawing presence. I couldn't seem to find the "why" to the ache of my heart which made the torment all the more intolerable and infuriating.

At least if I had been abused, or had a valid excuse, it could have been justified! Life all around was just splendid, and I was everything but dandy. Suffering that had meaning or cause seemed easier to endure and accept. How could I articulate my pain to others when I didn't even understand the source of my own suffering?

There were a few glimpses of joy when I actually felt alive, like when I would listen to music and especially my favourite band, Van Halen. They were like a shot of intravenous to my soul and made me feel naturally high. On the flip side, when I wanted to feed the darkness within me, I listened to Gregorian chants. When I hear those chants today, they make my skin crawl! Music was fuel to my soul and to this day, I find no easier way to enter God's tangible presence than through worship.

Another highpoint was playing trombone in our high school concert band with my dad as the conductor. That to me was one of the highlights and best memories of my life. It felt almost magical at times. If it weren't for my involvement in music and sports, I sincerely don't think I would have made it.

Then there was Rocky, my childhood hero! I loved that story of overcoming the odds no matter what. I would exercise while I watched his training scenes and had that soundtrack blasting daily. Maybe my favourite quote from him can inspire you as well:

"Let me tell you something you already know. The world ain't all sunshine and rainbows. It's a very mean and nasty place, and I don't care how tough you are it will beat you to your knees and keep you there permanently if you let it. You, me, or nobody is gonna hit as hard as life. But it ain't about how hard ya hit. It's about how hard you can get hit and keep moving forward. How much you can take and keep moving forward. That's how winning is done!"
—Sylvester Stallone, Rocky Balboa

Remember: Isolation Kills

If you have teens, I encourage you to make sure they are involved in some form of extra-curricular activities. You never know, it may be the one passion that will make them come alive and give them a sense of value and belonging.

Perhaps your teenager likes to spend time locked up in their room. There is nothing wrong with that in moderation, but if it is a daily thing and you have limited communication, I encourage you to open that door and make way for honest talk.

Usually, nothing good happens behind closed doors.

If my life sentence was to be tormented while on earth, then ending it myself seemed like the only solution or way out. Hopelessness is when we feel there is zero hope for change or improvement, ever. It's the feeling of "this is it for me," as though there will never be light at the end of the tunnel. But it is a lie and you do have a purpose and a future and there is hope for you.

The imposter in me was the bodyguard to my imprisoned and dying soul. My suicidal thoughts grew more insistent as my lack of nutrition caused my mental and overall health to decline. I couldn't figure out how to go through with it.

Apart from being an extreme sports junkie and a reckless driver at times, I never officially attempted suicide until grade 12. It wasn't a blatant attempt but one that now, looking back, was perhaps a little too close for comfort.

Every year our high school band would go on a trip, and in my senior year of high school, we did an exchange with a band from Austria. I was at an all-time low. I felt as though my world was getting smaller by the day as though I was caving in under my own darkness. Every day felt like an impossible uphill climb, and a losing fight for survival.

My life felt like a waste of space, and the light within me had grown increasingly dim.

The colours in the mountains of Austria were lush, and majestic. The richness of the landscape was breathtaking and jaw-dropping, to say the least. Sadly, I couldn't even enjoy them. It was as though I was watching a movie and it all felt so surreal and out of reach. Nothing felt real to me except for my pain and the constant heaviness that oppressed me. My ability to be in the present was robbed by my negative thoughts and constant obsession with my food intake or lack thereof.

My parents were on this trip. Dad was the band conductor, and Mom was one of the chaperones and I was billeted with a great Austrian family. If you know Austrian cooking, you can imagine that real sausage, cheese, and eggs for breakfast made for a highly unsettling experience for me as an anorexic!

We visited many interesting sites, castles, and even Mozart's home, but one day we went to the Auschwitz Concentration Camp. I don't even know where to start. Sobering. Humbling. Overwhelming. There was a cloud of heaviness over that place that was so thick you could almost cut through it. I know I wasn't the only one who felt it.

The camp, the gas chambers, the ovens. Even as I write, I am flooded with tears, recalling the day. I can't put into words what we saw, but I remember feeling this sense of guilt, like, "You think you are suffering? Get over yourself, Mel!" We can't even begin to fathom or comprehend what really went on in the concentration camps. And I will leave it at that.

All I can say is *thank you* to the soldiers who sacrificed their lives and limbs for our freedom, both then and those on the frontlines today.

May we NEVER forget.

Too Close for Comfort

One day, I went for my routine walk. It was late afternoon, and I remember the warmth of the sun hugging me. I was by myself, walking on a narrow road, through the lush rolling hills of Austria. I had climbed up a slightly steep hill and was on my way back down the other side.

I heard a car coming up behind me on the hill, so I knew it wasn't far. In that split moment, I made a deal with God. I was done. I basically told Him that IF He had a plan for me, He would spare my life. If not, He would take me home. Just like that, just that fast.

With my eyes closed, I stepped into the middle of that narrow road. Waiting for the car to take me out, I heard a screech. My heart was beating outside of my chest, and I felt a lump in my throat the size of a grapefruit. When I opened my eyes, the car was getting out of the ditch back onto the road and just kept driving ahead.

I burst into tears as I walked off the road into the field and sobbed under an oak tree. I was angry, scared, and I let God have it. "What do you want from me? Why am I here? You better make it clear because I can't do this anymore!" I wept and sobbed on my knees for what may have been 15 minutes, feeling as though my insides were coming out of me. My bones, ribs, and my entire body ached all over. I felt as though all my strength had been sucked out of me.

That was my first and last "conscious" suicide attempt. I believed He kept me alive for a purpose. My depression and suicidal thoughts were still very strong, but I didn't act on them. It wasn't until I was 28 that I was delivered from depression and suicide and apparently, I wasn't the only one suffering from it.

I've heard that suicide accounts for about a quarter of all deaths among teens and young adults. Apparently the stats are much worse in First Nations communities.

It's time we stop pussyfooting around and get real and raw with one another and especially our children. How many times have we known someone who committed suicide and everyone said, "I had no idea he/she was suffering!" Of course we didn't, because they were wearing *the mask*. That person didn't feel safe enough to reveal their true condition.

This problem can be prevented as long as we are willing to put an end to judgment and stigma and realise we are all fragile human beings who need one another to survive. Having raw, honest, and at times uncomfortable conversations can't be optional any longer.

The result of staying quiet can cost a life, and that is unacceptable. Whether it be your daughter, son, spouse, or friend, no one should ever slip through the cracks again! Somehow, society has created a culture where people feel safer being frauds than being vulnerable and authentic. It's high time we stop pretending and get real because we are all human beings on the same team called the human race.

"I would have despaired unless I had believed that I would
see the goodness of the Lord in the land of the living."
—Psalm 27:13

CHAPTER 3

Anorexia:
How Starvation Became My Voice

"Anorexia was a slow suicide, a way for me to tell the
world, 'Everything is *not* OK.'"
—Melanie Willard

Note: To *not* give fuel or ideas to anyone suffering from eating disorders, I will refrain from sharing numbers, habits, or any other shenanigans I entertained with this deadly disorder. Unfortunately for many anorexics, this disease is a warped competition. The winner is typically the sickest and thinnest, and I will not give an opportunity for that illness to gain momentum in anyone's life by sharing detailed rituals.

My depression and starvation just kept getting worse during my final year of high school. And even though I was barely eating, I never dropped a pound until I went to College in Ottawa. It became a relentless and all-consuming obsession. My social life, my relationships, my overall health, and brain functions all paid a terrible price.

I isolated myself from everyone and just wanted to die. To evaporate.

One of the few things I regret in my life was a decision I made in grade 12 when I opted to pursue fitness instead of music. I remember it like it was yesterday. I had just spent a week in an intensive countywide concert band called the Youth Band, which my dad had birthed years before. We were taught by professional musicians, and I loved every minute of it. I played the bass trombone, and my dream was to pursue music and play with the Canadian Armed Forces Band.

On the final night, we played a concert for the community. For some reason, I got a ride from a fellow band member, and I was sitting alone in the back seat, looking out the window at the pouring rain. It was at that very moment, and I even remember the exact location in Cornwall where I decided that I would not pursue music, but *fitness* instead.

Why, you ask? Because I was sick. Very sick.

I was afraid I'd lose *control* over my strict exercise and diet regimen and that all the hours of practice would cause me to gain weight. An anorexic's worst nightmare is losing control over what goes down their throat. I am convinced the disease made that decision for me. It felt almost traumatic, as though I couldn't fight back and Melanie was no longer in charge of Melanie, but this beast of control and self-hatred was. The moment I made that decision, something inside of me died.

I remember weeping and Melanie crying out for the imposter to make the right decision, but her voice would not be heard. I felt like I was in a prison cell crying out for anyone to see me caged up inside. Couldn't anyone see that deep down I wanted to pursue my number one passion, music? But no one heard my silent cry. I felt a lump in my chest. I'd been betrayed by my false self. The imposter was gaining strength and authority in my life, and the real Melanie had to bow down and obey. It infuriates me to think of just how bound I was to this dictator within me.

Motivating Factors

Many things contribute to a person developing an eating disorder, and one of the key ingredients for me was my obsession with Lent. Since I was all about being the perfect child in every way, I figured I had to sacrifice something to be more pleasing to God.

It was normal for our family to engage in some form of sacrifice during Lent, and it was usually food-related, like dessert or junk food. So for me to fast from television or something other than food never even crossed my mind. I remember being a pre-teen and jumping on the bandwagon. I would be "allowed" certain foods and not others because of my martyr-like sacrifice.

Having an addictive personality, I felt I needed to do more every year to be as acceptable. So the punishment and sacrifice grew more severe, and the rest is history. That was for me one of the biggest open doors to my "all or nothing thinking," especially the "good or evil" food syndrome. If I performed flawlessly I felt worthy of His love but if I failed, I was convinced He would withhold His love from me.

If I ate food that was on my "bad" list, then somehow *I was bad,* or *I was a failure.* If I ate "good" food, then somehow that made me more acceptable or pleasing. But this was the sad part. Once Lent ended, people would comment about my food saying, "YOU are eating dessert?" or "YOU are eating chips?" Instead of saying, "Yes I am," and telling them to piss off, I interpreted those remarks as rejection, judgment, and failure.

My identity was getting wrapped up in being a self-controlled fitness freak. I had to be perfect for God and others, and food was my way of performing flawlessly. Combine my all or nothing thinking, depression, perfectionistic and high-achieving personality, self-hatred, and distorted body image, I had the perfect recipe for a disordered eating disaster.

Although the average age of onset is 14, many girls start being preoccupied with their weight at an alarmingly young age.

Trust me when I say eating disorders are highly complex and much deeper than just skin deep.

As I mentioned before, I had three special friends in high school and two of them were aware of my struggle with my body and depression. I saw a school counsellor, but I felt like I was talking to a wall, and we just didn't click. So that was my first and last official session during high school.

My girlfriend recommended I talk to an adult whom I trusted, and it was then that I decided to reach out to a gym teacher and coach. This man soon became like a life coach to me, on and off the court. A mentor and friend whom I love and cherish and who continues to play a significant role in my life to this day.

Working with people who suffer from eating disorders is highly frustrating and demanding because there are so many factors that play into this disease. There is never an easy fix or solution, and most individuals will require professional help. There is little that can be said or done to help because the illness is so deeply fixated and ingrained in the person that it is difficult to change without digging into the root causes.

It wasn't until I went to college that the weight started falling off, and I mean falling off *fast*. Up until this point, the imposter had flawlessly hidden my true condition, but as the weight visibly peeled off, I could no longer deny the problem. I lost an alarming amount of weight and to this day I still don't know why the weight suddenly peeled off when I moved away.

This coach of mine worked with my dad at our school and was a friend of the family. So, once he felt my condition could no longer be kept between us, he spilt the beans to my parents. My secret was now in the open and my parents were devastated, to say the least.

My first year of college was one of the worst years of my entire life. I took Recreation Leadership in school while working about 25 hours per week. I rented a room in a home with a middle-aged single woman with a cat. That was one decision I still regret. I had the option to move in with two friends, but my illness always made me choose isolation over company. In my opinion, cats didn't belong on kitchen counters and that cat had free reign to go wherever it pleased in the house.

Until one day.

That dreaded day, it decided to pay my room a visit. Now, since I wasn't emotionally stable and pent up with rage, I walked into my room shut the door behind me. I kicked that cat like it was a soccer ball and it went flying up in the air, hitting the wall and with its four legs spread out, screeching as only whiny cats do! *Reeeeeeoooooooorw!* It's a visual I will never erase from my memory! It never made its way back to my room. I wonder why! This is not meant to traumatise you cat lovers out there, but to hopefully get a chuckle out of you.

I made a few great friends in college, and one girl stuck out from the rest. She was very compassionate, caring, and patient with me and my disorder. Throughout the course of my journey, I could see God's hand in my life, and one way

He did that was by bringing a person or two into my life when I needed it the most.

As I became more and more isolated, it felt as though my inner darkness was a bottomless pit. I could be in a crowd of people and still feel completely alone. My life as a whole was becoming more controlled and constricted. The dark world I created for myself was extremely small and suffocating. I was incapable of enjoying everyday life or relationships. All I wanted to do was hide, be invisible, and be by myself.

Around that same time, I was sent to the Eating Disorder Clinic at the Ottawa Hospital. I was an outpatient there twice a week for almost two years. I had one-on-ones with psychiatrists and psychologists and many group therapy sessions. As I look back, those group sessions sometimes did more harm than good because by sharing our habits and struggles we gave each other ideas. For this reason, I'm pretty sure that 20 years later the format has changed and improved.

I wanted to die, but because I promised God I wouldn't attempt suicide again, every pound I lost made me feel one step closer to my grave. Since I had never rebelled in high school or truly spoken my mind, this disease had officially become my voice. It was my way of revolting against my family, the world, and myself for not being ME.

Help!

It was my way of stating, "Hello! I'm not doing so well in here; can anyone hear me? Can anyone help me?"

This is why I am so deeply passionate about encouraging parents to *talk* to their kids even if they think they are doing fine. We need to be honest and open with each other and accepting of one another in all our differences and weaknesses!

It's not that my parents didn't want to be there for me. *I* never gave them a chance. The slightest hint that they didn't understand me was enough to shut me down. Because to me, being understood meant I was loved and accepted. On the flip side, for me to be misunderstood meant I was rejected and flawed—there was something wrong with me.

We don't all need to be the same or see life through the same lens! Can you imagine how boring that would be? If your kids are different from you, don't try to make them more like you. Accept them and help them grow in their unique strengths and qualities.

Even though Dad was gentle and sensitive, I didn't feel like I could talk to him. I didn't want to impose on his time since he was so dedicated to his music program at the school on top of his regular teaching schedule. Plus, he was a male, and I figured he wouldn't "get" me. And I felt that if he knew I wasn't happy, I would disappoint him and lose my perfect image.

Mom, on the other hand, was super positive all the time, stable, and never had PMS a day in her life. I felt we were far too different for her to get me. Her positivity is one of the qualities I most admire and appreciate in Mom today, but at the time I found it to be very irritating and superficial.

Heck, I didn't even understand what was going on inside me, how was I supposed to articulate it to others? All I could do was cry. Even in conversations at the dinner table or with friends, I always felt like my voice didn't matter. The minute I would try to speak up or join a conversation, I would be cut off or misunderstood. So I kept to myself. Instead of putting my foot down, speaking up, and commanding the stage, I shut down completely. Sadly, this muzzle silenced me until my early thirties.

My extreme sensitivity to men's looks was as strong as ever. However, I had finally erased all feminine curves and body parts. I developed early as a girl but never became plump. Some teased me, saying that I looked like two peas on an ironing board, but now I was more like two specks of salt. There was nothing left. I honestly looked like I was coming out of a concentration camp. I even purposefully slouched so that my woman parts would not show in any way.

This was what I was after, for men to no longer gawk at me or undress me with their filthy eyes.

I finally felt *invisible*.

I couldn't possibly care any less about my body, my appearance, or the clothes I was wearing. I often wore men's boxer shorts with a tank top. I wasn't a pretty sight. I had given up on myself, on life, and was just waiting for my time in this world to expire. Life was a blur, and school was difficult without my brain properly functioning. I don't recall one good memory from those two years. I would walk two hours to work, rain or shine, -30 °C or not. The more suffering I endured, the more vicious the whipping, the more pleased I was with myself.

I avoided eating in public like the plague because I felt all eyes in the restaurant were on me, judging me for eating. It was as though I could hear each person in the room loudly proclaim their thoughts in unison about me, "Look at her, why is *she* eating?" "What a failure," or "What a disgusting and fat pig!" It was sheer torment, as though the world was caving in on me.

Imagine for a minute that the only thoughts to preoccupy your head are about food. Or maybe it is sex, or drugs, or shopping for you. We always want what we can't have. Once something is forbidden, it becomes like an insatiable obsession because it is "off limits" or unattainable. From my first thought before I crawled out of bed to my last before I fell asleep, food held my mind hostage.

The Horrendous Side Effects

I started growing a thin carpet of hair all over my body, and I lost my period. When a body loses too much weight, it thinks it is in survival mode and focuses its energy on maintaining the functioning of its major organs such as the heart and lungs. The menstrual cycle is not necessary for human survival, and so the body focuses its energy elsewhere. I felt cold all the time, and when I combed my hair, clumps would come out, like a cancer patient.

I had headaches galore, and when I was at my lowest point, my heartrate was down to 33 beats per minute. Over the years I had seven root canals and lost five teeth. The toothaches were so painful that I would have stuck a fork in my leg just to distract me from the pain. To this day, my stomach and digestive system are still affected. I had painful Irritable Bowel Syndrome for years.

Believe it or not, I love a good steak today. Especially bison and bear! Who woulda thunk 20 years ago that I would one day become a meat lover? So there is hope for you and your loved ones!

In the beginning, my struggle was partially about the weight and my intense self-hatred. But as the disorder deepened, my weight started to drop to the point where the numbers didn't matter, nor did the look. It was a slow suicide. Even when I looked like I came out of a concentration camp, that didn't matter. I didn't even see it. I felt as though I were already dead.

My body was the shell driving around a dead soul and the vehicle through which I voiced my cry.

Here is a side note for you and the women in your life.

Just because a woman is not emaciated doesn't mean she isn't struggling. Many bulimics are at an average weight and to the untrained eye, it can be very difficult to identify a problem. Having been there, I can spot a struggle in someone fairly easily. However, like any other addict, most will deny it to the death.

Whether someone is male or female, try not to comment on their weight loss or gain. If they gained, they may feel like a failure. If they lost, it will only fuel their mission. Instead, ask them how their life is overall.

I remember I messed up big-time about six years ago when I spoke with an anorexic. I told her she looked healthier than the last time I saw her. I knew right away what was likely going through her head. Trying to cover my tracks, I went on to explain she had looked sick and emaciated and she was way more beautiful and attractive now. But I knew better. Why did that spill out? I still kick myself for that one. She *wanted* to look sick and overly skinny.

Another piece of advice: do not comment on how much or little people are eating, especially anorexics. During my recovery, I remember eating a cup of pasta. I told two friends from college, and one person said, "Wow that is great," so I felt like I failed because success only comes by *not* eating. And the other said, "That's it?" and then I felt like no matter what I did it wasn't good enough. No matter what is said to an anorexic girl, I guarantee it will get twisted. Everything becomes distorted in their minds.

All this to say, many individuals struggle with their body image and relationship with food. Bite your tongue, and don't say anything.

Men can also obsess with their body image! Some feel fat and insecure so they pick on the slimmer guys. Others are skinny and will go as far as injecting steroids to put on size. Society has determined what is acceptable and fashionable and because of that most of us struggle from low self-esteem, even those who meet the so called *standard*.

Let's be kind to one another. If you don't have something good to say, don't say anything at all because life and death are in the power of the tongue. And I think life is challenging enough without adding salt to a wound. We should always look to bless, encourage, and uplift everyone we come in contact with.

Cyber Competition

I firmly believe that what is more toxic than the fashion world today is the cyber world: the issue of porn in our society. Not only does it cause damage to relationships but it also harms a woman's self-esteem. The average woman does not look and cannot compete with your typical porn star.

When men frequently entertain these images, eventually the real deal doesn't stimulate quite the same. The woman constantly feels inferior and like she can never measure up or perform like her cyber competition. Now, I am not saying only men watch porn because I know plenty of women who do.

A porn addict is no different from a cocaine addict; both addictions involve the same dopamine receptors. The addiction physically rewires the brain, causing it always to want more and need more extreme stimulation to satisfy, just like cocaine. I doubt any of us who have watched porn felt a sense of accomplishment and pride when we closed our laptops. "Yes, that was time well spent!" Instead, most feel shame, guilt, loneliness, and a deep emptiness inside. And again, where do people usually watch porn?

Alone, behind closed doors, with the secrecy and shame holding them hostage to it.

In general (because we are on the topic of women's self-esteem right now), I don't think men would appreciate us going online to indulge in another guy's "package." We don't hear of men enhancing their private parts, yet I don't think there is one body part that a woman can't get altered! It has all become so normal that we don't even realise how ridiculously excessive it is!

Can you imagine telling someone from 50 or 100 years ago that we were going to give them a perky bum by injecting their stomach fat into it? Where do we draw the line? But that is the problem with humanity. We take everything to extremes, and we twist and alter what was once pure and natural. Deep down, most of us believe we are flawed.

Today fat pouty lips are *sexy*, and perky booties are in, but in ten years, skinny bums and thin lips may be the new fad. What may start as an innocent desire for improvement has the potential to become an obsession that will never be satisfied.

Whenever we do something to make ourselves feel better because of our "lack" in some way, that lack does not go away after we "fix" it. Instead, we find something else that needs fixing. Sadly, cosmetic and plastic surgeries have become multi-billion dollar industries today. I could think of a few places where that money could be spent more wisely.

I am not bashing or judging anyone who has had these procedures done. It is a personal choice, and I respect that. God only knows I have entertained the thought of getting Botox for the wrinkle party on my face! But knowing me, I would get hooked because most of these procedures only produce temporary results. Since I reached my 40s, I am working on accepting my wrinkles as a map of my life story for the world to read.

Ladies, true beauty radiates from the inside out and no amount of makeup can cover an ugly heart.

The Day I Thought Heaven was Calling my Name

Toward the end of my second semester, I was walking home from college exhausted and weak as always. I cut through the football field when my upper body went numb, and I felt a sharp pain in my heart. I dropped to the ground and thought for sure that this was it.

My chest hurt and I felt two more sharp pains. I lay there waiting and wondering what would happen next. It was as if the football field was spinning in slow motion. I was looking at the grass around me, and I honestly thought that I was about to breathe my last breath. Seconds later, once the pains had passed and after crying a few tears, I got back up and walked the rest of the way home. That was a real flirt with death and I was worried. But apparently, it was not my time.

I never told a soul (until now).

Then there was the time in my rented room where I was listening to the soundtrack from *The Mission*, and I was drenched with tears. I remember wailing and crying out loud with my mouth wide open when I saw two or three black clouds come out of me. They went up to the ceiling and vanished. It was like a black blob, or an entity, kind of like in the movie *Ghostbusters*. They were fairly big in size, maybe 12x14 inches, but void of any shape. I think a couple of dark spirits came out of me that day.

I thought to myself, "Hasta la vista, baby." Good riddance, and don't come back!

Alcatraz

Since I was staying at an alarmingly low weight, my doctor sent me to Toronto to look at the dreaded "inpatient" program. I was given two weeks to put on weight or else I was going to the anorexic jailhouse. When patients get to the point of life and death, the inpatient program is the last resort.

Since I wasn't doing the work on my own to get better, it would be forced upon me. And for the most part, before you can actually help serious cases you need to *feed* them first so that their minds can function. Otherwise, you are wasting time, and you likely won't get anywhere.

It's impossible for the body to snap out of depression if it is completely depleted of nutrients. So, in their attempt to give me a wake-up call, they introduced me to Alcatraz, the kingpin of all prisons for anorexics. They showed me the kitchen and dining area and listed all the foods that would be forced into me. That was all the wake-up call I needed. There was *no way* in hell anyone would tube feed me or force feed me in any way. My only option was to start making progress on my own.

It was then that I started seeing a family doctor who practised hypnotherapy. He had huge success with people trying to overcome addictions. It was kind of like behavioural hypnotherapy. I figured I would give it a try. Toronto was *not* an option for me, and I had two weeks to prove myself and put on a couple of pounds. The minute I regressed, I would be sent to Toronto.

My back was against the wall.

I had a lot of therapy over the years. My hypnotherapist helped me tremendously. I was also determined to do this *my* way because I was a stubborn control freak. If I was going to start eating again, it had to be on my terms and no one else's!

So, I began my gradual climb back to "health." Another thing that helped me greatly was that I got out of that cat-infested dungeon and moved in with two friends from school during my second year. A social life was forced upon me, simply because I was around others. This is why we can't let our loved ones isolate themselves.

ISOLATION KILLS!

I was around normal people who led normal lives. Plus, one of my roommates was a total goof and clown, and there was no shortage of laughter in the apartment. We played pranks on one another, and just being around someone who was so laid-back and happy-go-lucky rubbed off on me for the better. His friendship was extremely healing for me. He had zero masks and no pretences. He had nothing to prove to anyone, a "take me or leave me" type of attitude.

Although my grades dropped that year, in a way, it was a good thing. His example allowed me to stop striving for perfection and just chill! To this day, I smile every time I think of my roommate, and I am sure he has no idea the impact he had on my life.

Do not belittle your influence in someone's life no matter how *useless* you may feel. Sometimes making someone laugh is enough. It's not rocket science. You have no idea how much *you* can touch and impact someone by just being present and being yourself.

Although my eating disorder was losing its grip, my self-esteem had not improved. I still hated (and I *mean* hated) myself. Therapy helped identify origins for my disorder, but it only addressed the familial, emotional, and psychological causes. I knew there was more that had yet to be explored.

I strongly believe that in order for someone to be free, regardless of the issue or addiction, they must look at *all* aspects of their being by addressing the emotional, psychological, physical, and *spiritual* facets.

Unfortunately, this was round 1 for me in the ring with eating disorders.

Once I graduated from college and finished my treatments at the hospital, I was on my own and ready to face the world. I was doing OK overall, but I still controlled my exercise regime and food intake. I was living a fairly calculated life although I was much freer than ever before.

The thoughts occupying my mind were mainly about my weight, but at least I was eating fairly well. Perhaps this is the condition of most women today. Nothing overboard, but always preoccupied with nagging thoughts about their food consumption, competition with other women, and obvious body image issues. The doctors told me there was little chance of ever fully recovering from this disorder. But I remember telling myself, "No way! Sorry, but I refuse to believe that. I can't imagine living like this for the rest of my life, so I am not going to." I rejected that narrative as my future reality. Twenty years later, I am a living testimony proving my doctors wrong!

But trust me, it didn't come without an all-out fight.

Over the course of my recovery, I had given up on the thought of becoming a fitness instructor because, to my mind, the whole scene was all about body image and the *outward* appearance. It felt shallow to me at the time, and so many people in that scene struggled with eating disorders. I didn't want to feed this vulnerability within me, so I got out.

You are perfect and beautiful. You lack no good thing. You are not a mistake and I pray these words of truth would penetrate every ounce of your being and silence the lies that say you are *not enough*.

> "You are altogether beautiful, my love;
> there is no flaw in you."
> —Song of Solomon 4:7

For now, off we go from the frying pan into the fire.

CHAPTER 4

Domestic Violence: Welcome to Hell

"Find someone who will leave you covered in kisses,
not covered in scars."
—Anonymous

In the fall of 1994, I went on an epic two-month adventure to North Carolina to become a certified mountain guide. I was twenty years old and decided to pursue my passion for the outdoors. I met many free and kindred spirits from all over the world! We fully immersed ourselves in every type of adventure: white water canoeing, hiking, climbing, and high ropes' courses. To me, that was the life!

As a team, we could easily be gone for weeks at a time in the bush, sleeping under the stars and washing up in the river. I was in my element and loved every minute! The Blue Ridge Mountains were breathtaking, inspiring, and fed my soul to the depths of my being. I smile just thinking about it!

When I got back to Ottawa that November, I got a job at one of the major outdoor equipment stores. Life was good and even though I knew this wouldn't be my career, it paid the bills at the time, and I loved the people I worked with.

One day in February 1995, I was invited to go to the Banff Mountain Film Festival since our company had free tickets. There was one guy there I didn't recognise, who was also on staff but hadn't worked in months because of an accident. He sat beside me. I didn't complain since he wasn't hard to look at.

When the film was over, we went to a coffee shop and chatted for hours. We talked about anything and everything. This guy was like no man I had ever met. He was far from typical or boring and had enough stories to write a book of his own even at 22.

He was intriguing, adventurous, charming, and mysterious, and pretty much had me at hello. Don't forget I was a sheltered goody two-shoes who had lived a clean and honest life until that point. Apart from my depression and eating disorder, I had it pretty good compared to most. I had never had a serious boyfriend or done drugs, and I was still a virgin (and proud of it).

Little did I know this man would end up taking me on a trip to hell.

A trip that I am still paying for today, and I'm not talking money. Ben was two and a half years older than I was, tall, blond, with golden or amber coloured eyes. He was an adventurous free spirit, who had a magnetic personality. He was a philosopher at heart, always thinking deeply and profoundly about life. Like me, he was a spiritual man on a quest to find God and in search of inner peace and freedom.

After a couple of coffee shop visits, I felt closer to Ben than I did with most of my dearest friends. He seemed so comfortable divulging his life story to me, and that gave me permission to do the same with him.

Ben's story was night-and-day different from mine. It was filled with abandonment, abuse in every sense of the word, and one traumatic event after another, a story that would make anyone cringe and end up in a mental institution.

He was born in Vancouver and grew up in Anahim Lake, BC. You need to get a visual for this place. The scenery was incredible! The village back then was made up of several aboriginal reservations all totalling a population of about 1000. There were two small general stores, one school, two churches, one RCMP (Royal Canadian Mounted Police) detachment, a restaurant, and a motel. There were dirt roads everywhere, and it felt like a scene out of an old western. I loved the remoteness of it and the simplicity of how the people lived. I remember feeling as though this community was stuck in a different era. This town existed and moved at its own pace and time.

A Horrifying Childhood

Ben was physically and mentally abused and tormented as a child. He was once beaten to a pulp as a young boy and thrown outside naked in -30c for hours. Eventually, his mother left, and he was taken from his home by social services and put into foster families at the age of nine. None of that was a walk in the park. He was sexually abused, and at one point was adopted by a gay couple who took pleasure in Ben also. The stories he had were like something out of a Stephen King novel. How could anyone survive and function after living through a nightmare like he did?

He was introduced to drugs around the age of ten, and a 40-year-old woman slept with him when he was 13 to give him lessons in the sack. So his high school years consisted of wild sex, drugs, and rock and roll. He could lure any girl he wanted with the seducing power he had about him.

He was also an adrenaline junkie, risking his life hang-gliding with equipment he knew was sketchy. He always said he had nine lives because of all the close calls he had with death. He was an extreme skier who never found a cliff too high or deadly that he didn't dare jump off. Impossible and dangerous were words that only fueled him to attempt the craziest of stunts.

He did not have his high school degree, nor did he have a job when we met, but I thought nothing of it. He was broke, but all these things seemed justified through his circumstances at the time.

Ben was a daredevil, and one unpredictable and crazy rebel that the wild and adventurous side of me was attracted to. You need to remember, up until this point when any "good" guy treated me right or with respect I pushed him away. I was unable to receive love because I didn't think I deserved it. I didn't love myself (yet).

Ben didn't treat me right, so it was perfect! He fed my self-hatred so I didn't have to hurt and reject myself any longer! It was his full-time job, and he did it impeccably.

Melanie was little miss Mother Theresa who was going to love him like no other. No matter what he did to me, I would not abandon him but stick with him through thick and thin. I would show him what pure unconditional love truly was for the first time in his life.

Looking back, that was pure, unconditional stupidity on my part.

I share these stories not to get an, "Oh, poor Mel," but with hopes of bringing awareness to a topic that doesn't get enough exposure. So many women are isolated and suffering quietly. Even if they wanted to leave, they couldn't because of the fear of retaliation or the price tag that could be their life.

I also need to add that Ben took his life in 2009, which is why I am able to share my story. If he was still alive today, I would *not* be writing this book.

Red Flag

The first red flag I saw was about three months into the relationship. I should have ended it then and there, but I didn't. Instead, my mission was to save this man.

He basically misinterpreted a comment I made, and for the first time, I saw him snap from normal to insane in a split second. His countenance changed, and his eyes went black. There was no soundness of mind left in him at this point. He just sounded crazy and was tearing into me like I had never experienced before. He pushed me around, pulled me across the room by my hair, and broke my front door.

All this over a petty comment about his cowboy hat! He made me feel like the worst person in the world. He was such a good manipulator that I even believed it was all my fault. He had a twisted way of putting shame and guilt on me and convincing me that I was in the wrong when in reality I was far from it.

No one with self-worth, self-love, and self-respect would ever put up with that type of insanity. That should have been my first and last encounter with his dark side, but sadly, it wasn't. I was all the more determined to show him what I was made of. My warped "saviour mentality" was going to save him from his hell. By the way ladies, this is impossible. Last time I checked, only one man claimed to be the Saviour of the world, and that wasn't you or me!

Stop trying to *change* or *save* your man.

Around that same time, he gave me an ultimatum that if I didn't sleep with him, he would have to "get some" on the side because Mr. Wonderful had needs!

I had always kept myself pure for my future husband. Old-fashioned, I know, but it was very important to me, and I wish I would have stuck to my guns. Until he came into the picture, I had many opportunities to jump in the sack with friends and strangers, but I was unwavering in my convictions.

At that point, even though I didn't want to give in, I thought I loved him enough to marry him one day, which made me feel justified to give in and bite his bait. Mr. Snake the king manipulator got his way yet again. It was one month before my 21st birthday.

One week later, he had another hissy fit for no valid reason and I came back from work to find that his stuff was gone. He had jumped on the next flight back to BC. I was devastated, to say the least. I remember sobbing on my brother's shoulder instead of thinking, "This guy is a nutbar, and good riddance!"

For the first time—my heart was broken.

I felt used, cheap, and in shock. Ben called me back a couple of days after he left and sang the song of, "Oh, I'm so sorry, I made a mistake and want you to move out here with me because I can't live without you." Thinking back, it makes me want to vomit. Oh, how I don't miss being so young, naïve, and vulnerable! That same week, I was offered a position as a Recreation Director at a resort in Northern Ontario. I was pretty easily convinced to move out West to the reserve with Ben, since my lifelong dream was to live in the mountains. So I had a decision to make.

Do I follow my brain which says, take the job up north? Or do I follow my heart for the first time in my life?

My conclusion was that if it didn't work out with Ben, I could always just come home and get another job. But if I didn't follow my heart, I might never find a love like that again! One of my friends from work warned me that he had been abusive to his ex. I appreciated his concern, but it went in one ear and out the other.

When I had something in my head, it was near impossible to convince me otherwise. I was like a bulldog, and you'd best get out of my way. I was all or nothing, and when I set my mind to something, I "got 'er done." One month later, I fit my entire world in my backpack and took the next flight to BC.

Welcome to Hell

When I arrived in Anahim Lake, my sheltered world—although not void of inner suffering—was about to be rocked and scarred for life. The day after I arrived, Ben confessed that he had cheated on me at the local rodeo. What do you think I did? Of course, I forgave him! Unfortunately, that was the first of *many* cheating episodes. More than my fingers can count.

The next three years consisted of torture in every sense of the word. We moved every three to six months because he couldn't keep a job if his life depended on it. Plus, he made enemies easier than he did friends. We would stay at people's houses until he had exhausted our welcome there.

We were isolated and alone.

I tried calling my parents on a weekly basis. His paranoia got the best of him, and he would often force me to speak to my parents in English because he didn't trust what I said to them in French. I had that imposter mask on so tight, pretending like everything was peachy, but in reality, my life was in shambles. Nobody had a clue about the monster I was living with.

In front of others, he was charming (for the most part). If I received letters or mail from friends, he destroyed them before I ever had the chance to open them. He controlled every relationship and interaction I had with people. He was hyper paranoid and did not trust me under any circumstance!

The First Major Gong Show

We ended up moving to Vancouver that fall because he got a job at a ski resort. One night we hit the town because he was unsettled and on the hunt for cocaine. We went to a few clubs and after some drinks and no "score" he was furious. We got in our VW van, and he totally lost it. He drove on the sidewalk, on the wrong side of the road with oncoming traffic, in downtown Vancouver—punching me the whole time.

One male pedestrian, whom he almost ran over, yelled at him to pick a fight with someone his own size. He then proceeded to take the curve on an off-ramp at about 100kms per hour, and I closed my eyes and asked for God to spare us. I thought I was going to puke, I was so scared and I was convinced I was going to meet my Maker. I think He heard my cry since I'm here to tell the tale.

After driving like a possessed man for a while, he just kicked me out of the van and left me there in the middle of God knows where. I think it was Surrey or Burnaby, but having lived there for only a couple of weeks, I had no idea where I was.

It was a long walk back to our place in West Vancouver, especially with a busted face, nausea, black eyes, dripping blood, and a dislocated rib. Luckily, taxi drivers were kind enough to give me rides as far as they were able to without charging me. I finally made it home about two hours later.

The next morning, he thought it was a good idea to "get it on!" Surely I was irresistible with my bruised face and nearly immobile body. The back/rib pain was excruciating, but he didn't seem to care. I remember lying there, looking out the window with tears streaming down my face.

The Insanity of Jealousy

Throughout our relationship Ben revealed the extreme insanity of his jealousy and all the rules that came with it. One day, driving down Robson Street a busy shopping area in Vancouver, I did the unpardonable. I accidentally looked out the window where two men happened to be walking.

The fact that they were male was the nail in the coffin. Ben snapped and yelled at me for "checking them out." He hit me, opened my passenger door, and kicked me out of the moving van. I tumbled onto the sidewalk and got a few scrapes. I got up right away out of embarrassment, and people kept walking and shopping as though nothing had happened. At the time, that was a good thing, since help from others would have potentially upset him further.

Looking back today, I am furious that witnesses did nothing.

Come on, people! If we witness someone getting abused or mistreated, I think it's our responsibility to step in and help. And if you are scared of the perpetrator then at least *ask* for help! Don't pretend it isn't happening because that beating may cost someone their life.

I wasn't allowed to look at anyone. Ben, on the other hand, was a pervert. He would go to strip clubs, was addicted to pornography, and whenever he was attracted to a girl, he flirted with her as though I wasn't even there. He would tell me what he would do with them in bed or what body part he was picturing naked. Plus a heck of a lot more that I won't get into.

He convinced me that all men thought the same towards women but that most men didn't have the balls to admit it. Women were pieces of meat to be devoured and sexual objects to be conquered. Now, considering that I was already uncomfortably sensitive to lustful men, this gave my dangerously low self-esteem a serious pounding.

I became tormented and paranoid of every attractive woman out there. I found myself comparing my goods with other women and being severely threatened by their good looks. It was as though their beauty cancelled and nullified my own. He loved skinny blonds, while I was an athletic brunette. Every pretty girl became an opponent I had to compete with.

In my mind, I was always "less than," flawed, and never measured up. The negative and ridiculous self-talk is a battle that still haunts me to this day. I wish I could say I have arrived in this area, but the assault was so deep that I still find myself very raw and vulnerable whenever I am in public with my man. I am still healing from my perception of all men being scum when it comes to their animalistic view of women and sex. And that is OK because we are all works in progress, right? One day at a time.

I am not making excuses for Ben here, but he had been hurt, lied to, and abused so much that it was impossible for him to trust me at all or anyone else for that matter.

Back to Civilization

At one point, he left to work in the oil fields of Northern Alberta for a month to make some real money. We moved from our last place to a new city to start over *again*. This time, we picked Edmonton. Mr. Wonderful was so sweet that he found us an apartment. He paid the first and last month's rent, which totalled $600.00, but forgot to mention what he had done with his fat $5,000 paycheck. I walked through the door of our very humble apartment, and it was empty.

Zero furniture. Zero money.

He had blown it all on strip clubs, booze, drugs, a new sleeping bag, and hiking boots. Being his thoughtful and generous self, he gave me a bracelet he bought for $2 from a vendor down the street.

My heart sank.

Here we were, both jobless, moneyless, practically homeless, but at least we had a roof over our heads, right? I'd say one-third of our relationship we were forced to live in our van. He never got a job for the three months we lived there, and I wasn't raking in the dough waitressing lunches at a Greek restaurant.

You can imagine what it was like when he would come to the restaurant and I had to serve people! If a table included men, I couldn't even look at them. This proved to be a challenge in the customer service industry! It was so bad, and I feared Ben so much, that even if he wasn't there, I still feared him. I was paranoid that he would show up while I was smiling at a customer or that he would watch me from a distance. It was almost as if his spirit or shadow haunted me, and I was paralysed in fear whether he was physically present or not.

Even as I write right now, my chest feels like it's closing in on me, and I'm having a hard time breathing.

Over the course of our relationship, I was introduced to pot, acid and mushrooms, but I wasn't a fan. I was somewhat curious about drugs, but I know for a fact that I would never have touched them, had I not been with Ben. You may have heard it said before that bad company corrupts good character.

How true! We become who we hang around. And without a solid foundation of confidence and identity in who we are, we will crumble under pressure. I realise my fear of Ben was a big reason why I gave in.

I want to talk to teens right now. If one night your friends thought it would be cool to jump off a cliff, would you do it? Probably not, right? Drugs are no different. And trust me, it's much better to be a leader and go against the grain than to compromise who you are just to fit in. Do not be afraid to stand up for what you believe in. If they don't respect you for it, they were never your friends to begin with. Just because something is on-trend doesn't mean you have to join in. Plus the harsh truth these days is that most drugs are laced with deadly chemicals and it is simply not worth the risk.

One night, Ben was on the hunt for cocaine but could not score. He had to settle for acid which is a hallucinogenic drug, in other words, you "see" stuff. We both took the hit and started drinking. I remember seeing all kinds of crap, but what stuck out to me were the demons I saw in the bar.

Some were hanging on the light fixtures attached to the walls while another was hanging on a chandelier in the middle of the room. At one point I went to the ladies' room. While I was washing my hands, I looked up at the mirror and saw this skeletal demon face staring right at me, like the ones I mentioned seeing as a child. My face was no longer my own but of that entity.

I remember thinking, "Is this what I've become? A walking dead woman?" That crazy trip resulted in a very messed up night that ended at 7:00 a.m. the following morning. The next day I took a walk and felt so dirty and gross that all I wanted to do was *cleanse* myself. But I didn't know how. I happened to walk by an outdoor community pool, climbed over the fence and jumped in fully clothed. I felt just as dirty coming out.

Forgiveness is a spiritual experience that no amount of physical water can cleanse.

Stranded

One time I accidentally smiled and said, "Thank you," to the cashier of a 7/11 who looked like a sumo wrestler, and Ben lost it. He left me there for two hours while I sat and waited for him on the sidewalk. I felt pretty stupid, but boy, I regretted saying hello and being such a "flirt" with the sumo man! Oh yeah, my mission was to get in his pants! Not!

I can't even count the number of times he abandoned me because of his tantrums. One time while we were living in Edmonton, he packed my bags and kicked me out of our apartment. I had a co-worker offer his home to me if I ever needed a safe place to go to, but I knew better than to accept help *especially* from a male. All the women shelters in the city were full, so I went to the youth hostel instead. It cost me $13.00 for one night for a space that accommodated eight people per room. Since Ben always took my money, I was left with $1.13 for dinner. I splurged on a banana, small yogurt and approximately ten pretzels from the bulk section. That was fine dining at its best! The following day, he came to my work as though nothing had happened.

One day while we were living in Anahim Lake, we were at least 25kms from town, and he lost it for a reason I can't remember. So, in Ben-like fashion, he kicked me out of the van. This time, I wasn't going to wait for him as I was in the middle of a logging road with zero traffic and trees on both sides. My biggest concern was the fact that this was bear infested territory.

So I trekked along, and boy was I ever thankful for my tree trunk legs that day! It was a scorcher, and I was wearing sandals and had nothing on me, not even water. A couple of pickup trucks went by, but I knew better than to ask for a ride from anyone. I walked and ran all the way back in three hours and fifteen minutes. I was so proud of myself for making such good time, but Ben didn't share my joy. He thought it was impossible and was convinced that I had hitched a ride. So out came the jealous monster with his whip and interrogation session.

Finally, it was our last night in Edmonton. We had just left our apartment and were getting ready to drive for four hours to our future home in Canmore. It was around 11:00 pm, he was in one of his moods and kicked me out of the car. Here I was alone at night in a park with *nothing*. I sat there on the curb wondering if he was ever going to come back. I figured the best chances of seeing him again was to stay put. Three hours went by as I nearly froze to death until I saw him pull up and yell at me to get in. I can't say I was relieved but I guess it was better than sleeping on that curb.

What had my life come to? At the time I knew it was wrong, but I didn't think I deserved better. Every day was a test of survival, and for me to even contemplate leaving required too much thought and energy.

By the way, next time you see a homeless person, remember they too are human beings who are worthy of love and respect. We *all* have a story. Be slow to judge and quick to love.

Walking on Eggshells

His controlling ways were inconceivable. I could no longer look anyone in the eye, and I couldn't look outside the car window if we were in a populated area. I was not allowed to be nice or friendly to the opposite sex, *ever*. I lived the rest of our relationship looking down which felt like a prison. It was emotionally and physically suffocating, and I was completely and utterly frozen in fear. One of the worst parts was never knowing who would walk into the house—the "good/normal" Ben or the insane madman. To say I walked on eggshells and was on edge 24/7 is an absolute understatement.

Lost in Paradise

We planned to go hiking for three weeks in the glorious and bear-infested Rainbow Mountains. Mr. Invincible didn't think it was necessary to tell park rangers where we were going (which is a safety rule). He refused to pack a map or compass. So we hitched a ride to a trailhead and started trekking with 75 lbs on our backs. After the first day, we ended up dumping some of our food because our packs were just too heavy for the intense and uphill climb. The view was a breathtaking and spectacular landscape, and the first couple of days went rather smoothly.

Not a day went by that we didn't see or hear a bear or its fresh smoking dung, but thankfully, our encounters remained civil. By day three, we were up past the tree line, and I remember hearing what sounded like a thunderclap or oncoming train. We looked down into the valley where a massive herd of elk were running in all their glory. That was worth the trip right there! My heart was pounding out of my chest, and I remember thanking God for the privilege of witnessing such a spectacular show. It was nature in its most uninhibited, rawest form.

Unfortunately, by day three, the trail got weaker and weaker, and the guideposts (cairns or inuksuks used by the Inuit to act as navigation tools, guides, and message posts) were fewer and fewer as we went along.

We were lost.

We spent the next nine days trying to find our way back home. You need to understand how vast this terrain was! Mountain ranges on every side, and apart from the one dirt road which was Hwy 20, we could have said goodbye to civilization for good. Had an accident happened, we would have been totally screwed. On that third day, we got in a fight and it was so bad he packed his stuff and sprinted down the mountain on very steep and rocky terrain.

He was done with me and wanted to leave me there to rot.

He did his best to lose me but I miraculously managed to keep up with him. He eventually got over it, but at this point, we had just run down a couple of thousand feet of terrain into a valley, where there was no sign of any possible trail. If we were lost before, then we had just entered oblivion. We were beyond turned around. Any hope of finding familiar terrain or landmarks was a pipe dream at this point.

So we wandered aimlessly for about eight days until we recognised the landscape around us. It took us about two days to make our way back to the road where we hitched a ride home. He thought it was funny, and after the fact, his dad told us the trail we had taken was indeed an old abandoned trail. Apparently, we were way off from the trailhead Ben "thought" we were on.

Needless to say, looking back, I hate myself for putting up with all his crap and for not standing up for myself no matter how dangerous that may have been. I was always doing things that put my life at risk. I was no longer my own person. I was his puppet.

I compromised my values and principles all the time, out of fear for my safety if I disagreed.

The man obviously had serious issues. Although never diagnosed, I believe he was a psychopath and sociopath with an extreme case of bipolar disorder amongst other things. He would go on spending sprees, always seeking the next high, while moments later he was ready to kill himself. He was addicted to sex and was a constant emotional yo-yo.

He would threaten to leave all the time and the next minute tell me he couldn't live without me. His nine lives caused him to develop a sense of grandiose, like he was invincible and destined for absolute greatness. He was a dreamer but never completed a thing in life. The minute he faced opposition, it was game over.

It was exhausting, to say the least.

Physical vs. Emotional Scars

I need to take a pause and underline the life-altering impact that verbal abuse can have on a person. Verbal abuse is much more common than people care to admit. The trauma can even rewire our brain and leave us changed forever. Yes, every relationship has its ups and downs, and no one is perfect. We all say things we regret, but consistent verbal assaults are unacceptable. These hidden scars are equally if not more painful than the physical ones and just as damaging to a person's soul.

Since physical wounds are *visible*, we usually get medical attention for them, and they tend to heal naturally. However, emotional scars are *invisible*, so we don't get them looked at. Rather, we walk around broken-hearted with wounds that never fully heal. The toxicity eats away at us until our hearts can no longer recover. Addiction and depression await the wounded soul.

> "Jesus spoke as if we are all broken hearted. We would do
> well to trust His perspective on this."
> —John Eldredge

Ben's verbal diarrhea was straight from the pit of hell. So much so, that any speck of self-esteem that I had built up over time was completely annihilated. I felt like I was worth less than manure in a pigsty. Any ounce of self-love or feeling beautiful in any way was completely destroyed and trampled on.

He diminished me to a pulp *with his words.*

He had me believing that I couldn't live without him, that I would never amount to anything and that I was a total piece of sh*t (to put it *very* nicely). The colourful language that came out of him I would never dare put on paper. So I'm just going to leave it at that.

If you are in a relationship that is verbally abusive, I want to counter those lies and remind you today that you do not need to believe them any longer. You are beautiful, brilliant, and perfect just the way you are. You bring value to this world, and you have a destiny that you alone can fulfil.

You are worthy of love and deserve to be cherished. Anything contrary to that is a FAT *lie.*

How About Some Peas with that Melon?

One day in Edmonton, I can't recall the horrible thing I did to deserve this pounding (as if our actions would ever validate a beating), but Ben completely lost it. All our belongings were destroyed (the little we had), holes punched in the wall, and my head beaten until it was honestly the size of a melon. I am not kidding. My eyes were black and almost completely shut. I looked like Rocky in the ninth round. I was all forehead, and you could no longer see my face structure at all.

I am not exaggerating when I say I looked like the face in the movie *The Mask* with Cher.

I must have gone unconscious from the concussion because when I woke up, he was going hard at it inside me and there was a bag of frozen peas on my forehead. How kind of him to bring down my swelling! I felt so weak afterwards. I looked at my face in the mirror with total disgust. It was like a scene out of a horror movie and it looked like a tornado had gone through our room. It never felt real (apart from the physical pain). I felt detached from reality and my surroundings.

I was obviously dissociating and in shock, as I didn't cry or shake, but I was numb all over, emotionally, mentally, and physically. I remember just being aware of my breath coming in and out. That was all that mattered at that point. Melanie was pretty much a goner.

A psychologist once told me that any man who forces himself on his partner after he assaults her is a psychopath. It's even worse if she is unconscious, as I was. I used to think that people in relationships didn't experience rape because they slept together all the time. But apparently, that's not the case.

What Was I Thinking?

Who buys frozen yogurt instead of ice cream?

At this point, we were living in Canmore, AB, a mountain town that should be on your bucket list to visit! We were living in a dungeon-like basement suite. The walls were a deep red colour. There was a dark presence—a heaviness—in that place that almost felt tangible.

It was 7:00 p.m. and we had a couple of drinks at the local pub. We argued about finances as we always did. He drove off in his usual tantrum, while I had to walk about 40 minutes. When I got home, I thought he had calmed down, but he asked for a bowl of ice cream. I told him to get it in the freezer, except I made the grave mistake of buying frozen yogurt instead of ice cream.

Surely, that mistake was enough to send anyone into a frenzy, right?

When he realised this, he lost it, and snapped. The bucket of yogurt came flying at me; he started throwing dishes and eventually hammered eggs at me. I don't know if you've ever had the joy of having a dozen eggs drilled at you, but let me tell you, it hurts like a son of a gun. Like a charley horse times ten.

Now that I was covered in egg slime and shells, I locked myself in our bedroom. Although the window in the room was at ground-level, it was too high for me to climb through. I only had time to consider the window when Psycho bulldozed his way through the door. I was nauseous, and my heart was pounding out of my chest. I was frozen solid in fear, and I knew what was coming.

In his rage, his eyes turned black.

That night he was wearing steel toe boots which felt like cement blocks pounding my skull. There are no words to describe the sound that made in my head. This resulted in a broken nose, two black eyes, and another concussion to add to my collection. The pain was unbearable, and I blacked out. Later on, Ben told me that he thought he had killed me. Apparently, my body laid limp on the floor, and he couldn't see me breathing.

So he went in the living room, sat on the couch, and contemplated what he would do with my body.

Once I regained consciousness, he threw me in the shower to clean off the eggs because he was taking me to the hospital. There was blood, egg whites, yolks, and shells everywhere. I thought I was going to puke and was extremely dizzy. I could barely stand up without falling over, so he had to hold me up while I was in the shower.

In a rage, he drove me to Canmore hospital where we were greeted by a nurse whom Ben didn't care for. He started yelling at her and almost punched her. She kicked us out of the hospital within minutes. We jumped back into his truck where he drove to Banff hospital about 20 minutes away. The nurse from Canmore had called them to let them know we were likely on our way, so we had police escorts waiting for us inside the front doors.

We were immediately separated, and I was placed in a secured room with a nurse. I stuttered every word. I froze and was so gripped with fear that I couldn't even feel my physical pain.

I could not stop crying or shaking.

One thing I do remember was the nurse. She never said much; she just cared for me. She held my hand, stroked my hair, and just sat with me. To this day, I remember her.

We can never underestimate the power of our presence in people's lives!

When people experience a crisis, you may feel helpless or powerless, but know that sometimes all someone needs is for you to be there and to be quiet *with* them. It is often our connection with people that heals and not necessarily what we say.

Two days later, I had surgery for my broken nose. Upon my release from the hospital, a nurse gave me a ride home to Canmore. When I got there, Ben was waiting for me. Unlike many abusive men, there was never a "honeymoon" stage.

He never apologised or felt sorry for what he did. *Ever.*

That morning he was in a bad space because he did not believe that the nurse gave me a ride home. I could tell it took everything in his power not to pounce on me like an animal again. He threw things and banged on the walls. I was holding on for dear life. Obviously still rattled from our episode, I was just trying to stay calm and make it through this moment alive. Internally and physically, I was shaking.

There was no rest or breather from the trauma and it just felt like one onslaught after another.

Sign on the Dotted Line

That same afternoon, he took me to a car dealership in town. He likely thought it was a good time for me to agree to sign for a truck he wanted. His timing to get his way was impeccable, plus he wrote the book on manipulation. Mr. Wonderful had no credit of course, so I had to put my name on that loan.

Everything in me was revolting and screaming inside.

So here was a $20,000 truck in *my* name that I wasn't even going to drive. I was silently protesting, "*Nooooo!*" and hoping the banker could pick up my eye signals that were dripping with fear. I didn't dare speak up because my next destination could very well have been the grave. I thought my two black eyes and obvious large white cast would have been enough to make the banker disapprove the loan. Work with me here, buddy!

Are you kidding me? Mr. Banker, did you not suspect anything was off? Really?

The very next day, I went to the bank alone and pleaded for the banker and the manager to take my name off that loan. Apparently, their hands were tied. Really? I have never worked for a financial institution before but shouldn't there be a system in place against such obvious *wrongs*?

I had a feeling this wasn't going to end well for me. And it didn't. The next year, he flipped the truck into a lake, and of course, he survived without a scratch.

And guess who was left with the payments?

When Justice Fails

Months later, we were in court for the concussion and broken nose episode, but unfortunately, the justice system (courts) failed me miserably. My pastor came to one of the hearings, as well as my victim services advocate. However, for some reason, there were a few other court dates where I had to go alone. Guess who came and sat right beside me in court and threatened to kill me if I testified against him!

I'm sorry, but that is messed up! How does that even happen? I was petrified and paralysed by fear.

The judge asked for my statement with Ben sitting right there beside me. He never asked about what happened or anything. He just asked what our plans were going to be moving forward.

STOP! What?

I answered the judge saying that we were going to work on our relationship and that Ben was going to work on his anger. What else was I supposed to say with my life on the line? Deep down I was crying out, "Doesn't anyone see something wrong with this picture?" Come on!

He got off with community service. What a joke.

Would I have needed to die in order for him to have been proven guilty? Again, Ben believed he was invincible, and once again, he was. He beat death. He was untouchable and apparently above the law.

It didn't matter where I was; he always knew where to find me. Even restraining orders were a complete joke. He would be waiting for me after work, hiding in the parking lot at night so I could never seem to escape him. I even had a friend of mine who was a retired police officer park on the side of the road in case Ben would be waiting. He was. My friend followed us from a distance, but Ben caught on in no time and lost him shortly after.

Once again, I found myself alone with him in the middle of nowhere. So much for the restraining order!

Had I tried to escape, he would have either chased me, run me over with his truck or given me another whipping. As a result, I felt like the systems in place were completely useless to me.

The Night I Drew the Line

Towards the end of our relationship, I was living with three friends in a beautiful old log house. Ben and I were taking a break. Well, at least he was since he had a couple of bimbos on the go.

Anyway, one spring night around 2:00 a.m., I was sleeping when all of a sudden I was woken up by a man breaking through my window. It was none other than Psycho himself. He was very drunk and maybe high. Who knows? I completely froze in fear. As human beings, we all have natural stress responses. Fight, flight, or freeze, and I was a "freezer." He put his hand over my mouth and threatened to kill me if I screamed. Having held a knife to my throat a couple of times, I believed he meant what he said.

The terror and psychological torment I experienced that night were unfathomable. I don't think words can adequately describe the horror I felt.

There was a shelving system in my room that had a cubicle-like hole, where he aggressively shoved and rolled me up into a ball just to fit me in.

He went on to tear every single piece of clothing I owned. He broke my stereo, CDs, and ripped my books to shreds. I remember seeing the Devil through his face and the pleasure he felt as he ripped each page. It was eerie, to say the least.

He proceeded to urinate all over me and the carpet like a total animal. Whippin' that thing around like it was a garden hose and his tongue sticking out. He was completely out of his mind.

Once he had nothing left to destroy, he grabbed me by the hair, ripped my clothes off, and you know the rest of the story. I lay there limp, numb, frozen—until he said to me, "This is what I will do to our kids because this is the only way I know how to love."

BAM! That was my wake-up call.

It was OK for him to hurt me because I didn't love myself, and didn't think I deserved better. But there was *no way* I was ever going to expose my future children to this insanity, terror, and abuse. Something rose up inside of me, and that was the last straw.

I remember laying there after everything was over and he'd passed out. I was looking at the door wanting to run for my life, but I was so paralysed I couldn't even get up to go to the washroom, let alone escape. My mind and spirit wanted to leave, but it was as though my body was pinned down by an invisible force. The force named *fear*.

It was a Sunday morning, and I finally escaped around 7:00 a.m. I found a couple of pieces of clothing that were presentable and cleaned up at the gas station. I went to church, and guess who was waiting for me after the service with his truck full of my belongings in garbage bags.

This is why we cannot turn a blind eye when we see or hear something suspicious.

I have received a lot of counselling, prayer, and deliverance in regard to this traumatic nightmare. I can still be triggered by some situations. However, I am patient and loving with myself through my healing process. I am very sensitive to confrontation and can be easily triggered watching movies, so I am selective with what I watch. I have come a long way in trusting my late and present husbands, but this too is a work in progress. All things considered, I think I have recovered fairly well. Thank you, Jesus.

You may wonder why I am sharing all these stories. You need to understand that after coming out of the storms of life that I have, if my story can help one girl to start loving herself and her body, or if I can help one person find hope to live another day, or if this can help one woman get out of an unhealthy relationship, then it will all have been worth it to me.

If you have lived through a traumatic experience in your life, remember:

- Having PTSD does NOT mean you are weak.
- PTSD may impact all aspects of your being.
- It can take a long time to heal and fully recover from it.
- It will not improve or go away on its own.
- Getting help is not a sign of weakness.
- Cut yourself some slack. After all, you are not Superman. You are *human*.

CHAPTER 5

A Surprise Encounter:
The Day Everything Changed

"He will redeem them from oppression and violence,
for their lives are precious to him."
—Psalm 72:14 NLT

Through all our struggles and moving from city to city, the one constant was that Ben and I were both on the hunt for God. We attended different places of worship and met pretty interesting people. It's not like we attended church every Sunday—far from it, actually—but we were searching nonetheless. Having grown up in a very traditional church setting, I was introduced to a more charismatic church in Anahim Lake. It was night and day different from anything I had ever experienced before and I loved it. I was on a quest for peace, freedom, and intimacy with the One my heart longed for!

Some people had their hands raised, others dancing, praying, or crying, and even though it was all taking place at the same time somehow it wasn't chaotic. Quite the opposite. Whenever the pastor would pray for me, it was as though he could see right through me. I would weep the entire time I received prayer and never felt safer than I did in those moments. Nothing was scripted or repetitious because it came from the heart and spirit rather than empty religion.

The thing that stood out the most to me was the presence I sensed in that place. I could feel the nearness of God somehow, and there was life! Trying to put this into words is a challenge, but that's the best way I can describe it. There was no confusion or striving at all. On the contrary, everyone was free to meet with God individually yet corporately. You were not told what to say or do. It was as though God was a welcomed guest and He was actually in charge of the service instead of "man." There was nothing boring, dead, dry or robotic. It was real, intimate, fun and free. Beautiful actually.

After seeking God my entire life, it finally felt like He was within reach. Seeds of hope were planted in me that God was as personable as I had wished Him to be. Apparently, I didn't need a priest or 100 Hail Marys to get through to Him either!

That was good news.

We would always end up meeting people who were willing to share their knowledge and experience of God with us. Sometimes I would chuckle at how He planted good people around us in the midst of our unstable and turbulent life.

About three years into our relationship, while living in that dungeon-looking basement in Canmore, I was at an all-time low. It was October 1997, and I felt like I couldn't keep living the life I was living. It felt as though this sinking and suffocating darkness was all around me and I was in a pit of despair. I was utterly hopeless that things would ever change. I think Ben was working that day (shocking, I know) and it was mid-afternoon when I collapsed to the ground. I wailed and wailed—unbearable groans that could not be uttered and that were far too deep to articulate. I was furious with God, and I let Him have it.

"God I've been seeking You and pursuing You my whole life. *If* you are the God of the universe, the creator of heaven and earth, and *if* You are who You say You are, then *surely* You can talk to me, touch me, and let me feel Your presence! So far, I've been banging my head against the wall with a one-way conversation hearing nothing from You! *If* nothing is impossible to You, then what's the problem?"

I was angry, and I was at the end of my rope.

It didn't make sense for a loving and all-powerful God to sit in Heaven and watch us like a puppet show on earth. I didn't believe He was distant and indifferent about our lives. Surely He created us for a reason, for a purpose. Otherwise, the stars and galaxies would have been fulfilling enough for Him! There was something in me that thought He created us to be intimate with us. And darn it, I wasn't going to settle for a life without Him in it.

I was NOT after "religion," I was after Him. His heart, His love, His presence.

I was after something that couldn't be scripted or rehearsed—something pure and completely unique and personal between Jesus and me. Something like any earthly relationship, but on a whole different plain.

That day, I wanted to die so bad, but couldn't think of how to go through with it. So my final words to God were,

"If *You* don't come meet me, then I'll go meet You."

The Day Everything Changed

About two weeks after my meltdown, we invited our pastor and his wife over for dinner (the first and last time we ever had guests over). We finished our meal, and our pastor used the restroom. Suddenly, I felt a warm presence hugging my entire being, as though a waterfall was washing over me. It was the safest, most beautiful feeling I had ever felt in my life.

I was a fountain of tears. It was as if the tap had been turned on and there was no off button.

When our pastor came back and saw me, he asked me why I was crying, and I didn't know. He then replied, "God is here." This lasted about two hours. For the first time in my life, I felt His tangible presence and no earthly thing compared to it! It was as real as the human touch. I was speechless.

I felt wholly and perfectly loved for the first time.

Nothing I could do or say could make Him love me more. Nothing could be added or taken away from that love; it was perfect and full and flooded my body, mind, soul, and spirit. I felt the weight of the world coming off my shoulders. That day when I asked, He was faithful to forgive me for all my mistakes and sins. I even *felt* forgiven, and the guilt and shame were no longer mine to carry. God spoke through my pastor that night, revealing things about me that only God knew.

God's promise to me, which meant *a lot* at the time, was from Jeremiah. God basically said that He had plans to prosper me and *not* to harm me, to give me peace, a hope, and a future. He went on to say that when I would call on Him, He would hear me and answer me, and that I would find Him when I pursued Him with all my heart.

That day, I found Him. The search was over, but the romance was only beginning!

You can imagine how His promise to prosper me and not to harm me was appealing. And He promised to give me peace as well? I had never experienced inward peace before. I felt as though God was reaching out to Ben as well, but he rejected Him. He sat there watching the show but was unable to receive it for himself. After our time had come to an end, my pastor and his wife left.

The moment they walked out the door, that split second, Ben's face was overcome with evil. His eyes turned black, and I thought to myself, "Here we go again." I thought he might be different after witnessing what just happened, but the opposite was true. It was as though the darkness inside him was protesting the event. Dishes went flying, and the kitchen table did a backflip. I don't remember how long Ben's hissy fit lasted, but at least this time he didn't touch me.

The End was Near

Our relationship continued for another eight months or so. Not much changed between us, except that I was different. I was changed and no longer able to take part in our lifestyle like I used to. I guess I was feeling convicted, like a small voice in me was tugging at my heart and saying, "This is wrong, and there is a better way." There was a genuine battle going on inside of me.

For the first time in our relationship, it was like my eyes were open to see how poorly he treated me. I could finally see just how sick and dysfunctional our relationship was. It was as if I was no longer "under his spell," but I had a newfound strength and boldness within. Even though I didn't act on it much, at least something was stirring within me.

That spring I got a job working for a National Park clearing trails and camp sites. You could say I was hiking for a living and getting paid for it. What's not to love about that? Ben was living in Canmore and scoping the "market" while I lived in Banff at the staff compound.

I was getting more and more acquainted with God and made incredible friendships at church. Their love and support were truly life-saving.

I was torn, since I couldn't live with Ben and didn't know if I could live without him. This just goes to show how toxic, unhealthy, and codependent we really were. Ben wanted us to bug off to Alaska or the Yukon to get as far away from all civilization as possible. I think he could sense he was about to lose me, and what better way to have me all to himself than by living out in the middle of nowhere? Part of that was appealing, as it was territory I would have loved to see. However, I knew deep down that if I left with him, I would never have come back alive.

For the first time, I had this sense in my gut that I would *not* live through it.

A friend of mine was visiting at the time, and I shared with her about my dilemma of moving up North. I also told her about the risks involved. Shortly thereafter, my parents got wind of my situation for the very first time in three and a half years. To say they were devastated, furious, and beside themselves is an understatement. My dad and brother's reactions were apparently the typical male protector responses. They all wanted to take the next flight to Alberta and give Ben a taste of his own vomit, if you know what I mean.

My parents came for a week, for moral support. My abuse was news to them, and obviously quite traumatic as well. I knew my parents were just a phone call away, but while I was in that situation, I couldn't seem to swallow my pride. Plus, I was on a mission to save Ben and for me to come home would have meant that I had failed.

A week later, I needed surgery (unrelated to Ben). I remember laying there in the hospital bed in Banff, and I heard a soft voice in my head say,

"Are you going to keep banging your head against the wall or are you going to follow Me?"

I believe Jesus spoke those words to me. He knows us and speaks to us in our language so that we actually get it! He doesn't want to confuse or trip us up. The lights went on, and something shifted inside of me. I finally built enough strength to end this gong show once and for all.

How it All Went Down was Nothing Short of a Miracle

It was a sunny spring day, and in normal fashion, Ben drove us out to a remote location in the middle of nowhere. You remember how terrified and paralysed I became due to fear? Well, this day was different. So very different!

> "Security is not found in the absence of danger,
> but in the presence of Jesus."
> —John Elderedge

Even though I was just getting to know God, I could feel His tangible presence and peace there. I had felt God on a personal level and at church, but I didn't realise God worked outside the church walls! I was in for a rude yet pleasant awakening! He wanted to be actively involved in all aspects of my life, as He was everywhere and never off duty. That was good news to me.

I basically told Ben how much he had hurt me over the years and that I couldn't live that way any longer. As I was always one to shrink back and weep during confrontations, it was really abnormal for me to have two very dry eyes. I kept my cool, but I had this boldness about me that wasn't my own! I had never seen Ben cry until that day, and he wept like a baby.

It was over. I called it quits. Hasta la vista, baby! The whole thing was surreal and the complete opposite of any interaction I had ever experienced with Ben. God was in the truck, and *God* was in charge. For the first time ever, I was fearless. *Wow!* That was a miracle in itself!

"You are my hiding place; you protect me from trouble.
You surround me with songs of deliverance."
—Psalm 32:7

Just writing about this now, I have tears of joy streaming down my face. Unlike popular belief, God is truly *good*. He is not this dead or distant God who lives in a building! He is real and cares more deeply about you and me than we could ever imagine. He knows us better than we know ourselves!

Another miracle was that Ben never pursued or stalked me after the breakup. He called me once to see if we could get back together, and I didn't flinch one bit. He was dead to me! Those chains were broken, and I was a free bird learning to fly with broken wings!

This experience revealed to me that God had my back, and He was on my side! I was His now, and He wasn't going to let anything or anyone hurt me any longer. It was like I could feel Him putting His foot down with and for me! My Defender, my Strength, and my Deliverer were all attributes of God that I discovered that day.

When we say yes to God, He makes His home in us. He promised to never leave us, and it is comforting to me to know that I am never alone no matter what. The more He revealed Himself to me, the more I wanted to know Him.

While the majority of us "know about" our prime minister, most of us don't know him intimately. We don't have dinner with him or anything, and the same goes with God. Many people know *about* God but don't have a personal relationship with Him.

Anything short of falling in love with our Creator is religion. And God **hates** religion.

It's a Divine Romance, Not Religion

I want to encourage you with this today: if your perception of God is anything other than Him being all loving, perfectly just, breathtakingly beautiful, recklessly pursuing you, and *good*, then you have an inaccurate picture of His nature.

Perhaps you suffered unfair blows in life, and blame God for them. Maybe you have been hurt by the church. Or maybe you've seen Jesus misrepresented through Christians like the crusaders, sexual assaults from priests, or the white man with First Nations and the African American peoples.

It's no wonder some people want nothing to do with Him! Heck, if any of those atrocities were done to me in the name of Jesus I'd want nothing to do with Him either. Trust me, God wasn't the source of any of it. Anything that is done "in the name of Jesus" but is so contrary to His character needs to be questioned. There is one being and his little minions who are working overtime to stop us from realising how good God is.

On behalf of Christians everywhere, if we have ever offended or mistreated you in any way, I am so deeply sorry. I hope that you will not let "man's" mistakes or inability to represent Jesus accurately rob you of intimacy with your Maker. He is so much better than we think! Erwin MacManus' words are unfortunately true:

"Jesus is being lost in a religion bearing His name."

I hope Jesus won't pay the price and be shunned by you because of our mistakes as Christians. The thought of that truly grieves my heart. He knows every single detail about you: the good, the bad, and the ugly! He loves you where you are at, and because of that same love, He won't leave you there. He will be involved in your life to the extent you want Him to be. Maybe you hear Him knocking at the door of your heart today.

Will you let Him in?

Think of a concert, for example. Jesus already paid the price and bought our ticket for us to attend. If we say yes to Him and go in, we get to choose our seats at that point. In other words, if Jesus is the singer on stage, you chose whether you will sit in the nosebleed section, on the floor at a comfortable distance, or better yet, if you will sit on His lap.

With Ben finally out of my life, I continued working for the Park and later on at a coffee shop until the New Year. During these months, I was seeing a psychologist to help me process my gong show. At the same time, I was getting counselling from my pastor and his wife. I remember that the sessions with my psychologist were about all the work and healing God was doing in me. He honestly felt like his impact was minimal compared to what God was doing, and that it was maybe time for us to part ways. My Doctor felt like he couldn't compete with God! We both concluded that I would just get counselling from my pastor, but the door remained open should I have needed him in the future.

A Memorable Visit

I remember one night, I was still living in Banff at the staff compound. My pastor and his wife were over for what ended up being a three-hour counselling session. These were unlike any other therapy sessions I had ever known. God (knowing me better than I know myself) would reveal things to them about me that only God and I knew.

Since I was ashamed of certain areas in my past, there were things I wasn't comfortable sharing and God knew that. But He trusted them with my heart and therefore revealed to them the things I kept hidden (like the day I tried "purifying" myself at the outdoor pool).

> "God wants you to be delivered from what you have done
> and from what has been done to you—both are equally
> important to Him."
> —Joyce Meyer

God did this not to expose or shame me, but with gentleness and love He healed and restored me from a guilty conscience and cleansed me from my filth. He helped me forgive myself from my haunting shadows.

FYI, all sins are equal to Him, and He died so that we wouldn't have to carry the weight of our shame and guilt. I quickly realised that *nothing* was hidden from God and that for me to pretend like I could hide my "ugliness" or imperfections from Him was a joke. As if I could play God for a fool.

Once the evening was over and my pastor and his wife left, I felt like I had lost 1000 lbs. My roommate was away, and I found myself alone in my apartment. Now, you may or may not have ever had this happen to you, but five minutes passed and I felt a sudden chill, like a cold presence *whooshing* through me. I had shivers all over, and I was gripped with fear. I knew what God's presence felt like and this was the total opposite.

In the past, I didn't know how to handle evil altercations, but for some reason, I felt like I couldn't just watch anymore but I had a role to play. There was a "spiritual" intruder in my home, and he wasn't welcome. I wanted to tell it where to go but didn't know how. Knowing this wasn't a physical fight, I figured I needed spiritual weapons to deal with it. What good would punching into space or grabbing a knife do?

So I sang a song with the name of Jesus in it. I said His name out loud a couple of times, and I kid you not, immediately that sensation left, and my peace was restored. *Bam!* Just like that! I started laughing and kept singing to thank Him for being so cool and for having my back. Again He was actively involved in my daily grind.

My Mini-Vacation

Around early September, I was offered the chance to go on a week-long adventure north of the Whistler Mountains in BC. The trip was sponsored by the government for women who were victims of abuse and diagnosed with PTSD. Obviously, I couldn't turn down a hiking trip! I met other wounded souls, and there was one woman in particular whose story I will never forget—she lost her six-month-old baby in the womb due to too many blows to her gut.

It was a time of introspection, healing, tears, and laughter. The scenery was once again out of this world. It was heaven on earth for me! One of the ladies from the crew offered me a job with their organization as a mountain guide (since I was already qualified with them).

However, during my time there, I felt a tug from God. Since I was a little girl, I always felt called to serve Him somehow. The only way I thought women could serve God was by becoming nuns. Those beliefs were quickly crushed as I realised we can all serve Him in our own way.

Finally, on this trip, I decided to follow my heart and spirit and pursue my "calling," whatever that was.

In January 1999, I attended a missionary school in Tyler, Texas. I was there for a year and loved every minute of it. I went through so much healing and restoration that year, it was an unforgettable and extraordinary experience.

My greatest revelation was that I no longer had to take the whip to punish myself for my mistakes and that His love and approval of me was not dependant on my perfect behaviour. It messed me up *good*.

The perfect Melanie no longer had to be the authority over my life. I was free to remove the mask and slowly became my authentic self. I could finally quit the game of pretending and put to death the people pleasing imposter! It wasn't an overnight thing but a process that God was faithful to walk me through over the years. God was no longer a tyrant waiting for me to mess up so that He could strike me down with lightning.

It was as though everything I was learning about God wasn't textbook knowledge but through experience on a very deep and personal level. Falling in love with God can be compared to falling in love with a human being. Except sweeter still. *Much,* much sweeter.

> "Run my dear, from anything that may not strengthen
> your precious budding wings."
> —Hafez

CHAPTER 6

A Fresh Start:
Learning to Fly with Broken Wings

"If we do not give our ache a voice it doesn't go away. It
becomes the undercurrent of our addictions."
—John Eldredge

Once I got back from my mission's school, I decided to
move back to my friends and faith community in Canmore. I got on a nonstop 50-hour Greyhound bus trip from
Ottawa to Canmore. I had used up all my savings for my mission trips, so I was technically starting back at square one with
nothing but a bucket to piss in.

My pastor graciously offered for me to live at our church
in exchange for my cleaning services. It was an old police station that had been transformed into a church, and I turned
a spare room into my bedroom. My bedroom consisted of a
mirror, a CD player, a curling iron, and I slept in my sleeping
bag on the floor.

Even though my life was brought down to the bare neces-
sities and basics of survival, there was a simplicity to it all that
I truly loved. With all honesty, I felt like the richest person on

earth. I never craved "more" or what the Joneses had. I was content, and I had peace as far as my outward reality was concerned. I felt like a queen.

I got around on my mountain bike, and I was free as a bird. I pretty much lived in the mountains by day and went back to my church hut to sleep at night. The best way I can describe this season is that it was like a honeymoon with Jesus. I'd never felt so close to Him, spoiled, and loved. I felt very much taken care of. Just a sweet and precious time. I will never forget that season as long as I live.

I was surrounded by amazing people both at my work and church. Life was good, and I was incredibly grateful! I started attending a young adult's event every Monday night that rocked my world. I danced, worshipped, cried, and met with God every time. One night, I saw a job opening at that church for a custodian position. I applied and got the job and within a month I moved to Calgary.

It was a bit of a culture shock going from a church of 50 to working at a church of about 1500 members. The place was rockin'. I spent the next four years vacuuming, washing floors, and cleaning toilets.

However, I was happier than a pig in mud.

I worked alone a lot of the time, and I remember feeling God so very near. I put worship music while I washed toilets and would find myself laying prostrate on the bathroom floor weeping because of His overwhelming presence. Bathroom floor or marble floor—when God shows up, nothing earthly matters or compares.

Everything around us grows strangely dim in comparison to His presence.

I made quality friendships over the years and lived with two great gals. I definitely felt like I belonged and even though I was a janitor, I felt like my contributions mattered. I was part of different ministry teams where I was able to help people find greater freedom and hope in their own lives. I've seen thousands of individuals set free from bondage before my eyes. It's no gimmick or fluff. When we are open to Him working in our lives, nothing is impossible, and the sky is the limit! Life was good, and I was happy.

However, there was still a very real battle raging within.

I sought help from a counsellor at our church who helped me walk through some thick and muddy waters. He was one of my two most effective counsellors I had the privilege of seeing. He was caring, sensitive, and compassionate and I felt very safe with him. He was sensitive to God's voice and leading which is why I believe he was so effective. I thank God for him to this day.

Haunted by Yesterday's Trauma

We don't always pick our battles, but we decide whether or not we will let them conquer us. Even though I was doing great in so many ways, I developed PTSD after leaving Ben. I was able to work hard and function very normally in life. However, my emotions were a hot mess, and I had yet to learn the skills of expressing myself and articulating my feelings.

Not long after I left Ben, I began coping with bulimia— a vicious and unforgiving cycle of self-sabotage. But like many other addicts (regardless of the "drug" of choice), the minute I found myself alone, I gave in because I couldn't handle the pain.

Isolation is a cold and deadly place, and it is an incubator for addictions.

I was fine with others and in public, but the minute I found myself alone I had no idea how to deal with the boiling pot stirring within me. My ever-present lack of self-expression forced me to resort to yet another unhealthy coping mechanism. The only way I could appease the storm within was to shove food down my throat, and push down my emotions into the basement of my soul. My voice had yet to be found. However, in order not to gain weight, I had no choice but to purge.

So the binge "appeased" and quieted the loud screams inside of me. The role of the purge was to *empty and cleanse* myself from the physical discomfort of the food, the emotions, the shame associated with my addiction.

The irony with bulimia for me was that there was never a sense of relief from the pain. At no point during the ritual did I ever feel better. On the contrary, I *hated* every single minute of it. It was quite bizarre when I think about it now. Before I binged, I felt a panic attack coming on, like I was losing control. But like so many addictions, the relief was minimal and temporary.

That is why I encourage people to be well surrounded when they are dealing with hurts or past traumas like I was. It honestly helps prevent an addiction from becoming all-consuming and life-threatening.

I've noticed a common thread over the years that no matter what coping mechanism I struggled with, that particular addiction always felt like the worst one out there. I was so ashamed of my own struggles. This is why I believe a sign of overcoming an addiction is when we can talk about our past struggles without shame or embarrassment. Kind of like I am doing through this book. If I was still battling any of my past demons, I guarantee you would not be reading this book right now. My mouth would still be muzzled.

The Steep Cost of Bulimia

One thing I hope you get out of this book is that there is *hope*. You *can* be free from what is holding you back, and you *can* have peace. I am a living miracle to testify that it is possible if you don't give up and pursue it with all your heart. Be tenacious and don't settle until you are totally free!

For all of you out there thinking this may be a good way of coping or maintaining your weight in life, it is *not*! Maybe you know or suspect someone who is struggling with their weight and self-esteem. Bulimia is unfortunately very hard to identify with the untrained eye because although women may fluctuate they generally stay at a *normal* weight.

In this season of my life, I had lots of counselling and prayer about the eating issue, about Ben, and just life in general. The effects of my puking were evident in my body. I was often very tired and weak and ended up losing five teeth. To this day I can't have my teeth cleaned because I have zero enamel left on those pearly whites.

I was still bound by my *all or nothing, good vs. evil* thinking towards food. I had unbearable stomach pain and cramps, and a hoarse throat as well as swelled up "chipmunk" cheeks.

I also remember the nagging feeling and *lies* in my head when I would attempt to eat a normal meal. If I was with others, it wasn't as bad. But the minute I ate alone at home and promised myself to keep the food down, the mental torment and lies would begin flooding my mind. I felt "dirty" and like a failure for eating and so I figured I might as well pig out and just puke it out after. Because in my opinion, I had already failed.

It was impossible to let the food just *sit* inside me.

Sometimes I would do this two to three times in a row, each time thinking, "*No*, I can do this." But when I was alone, the food rarely got the opportunity to rest in my belly. It was a vicious cycle, to say the least. Over the years, I have counselled many women who have admitted those same thoughts and struggles. The language is universal. Unfortunately, this disorder is much more common that we all realise. By the way, many bulimics were victims of abuse and especially sexual abuse growing up. Hence the need to suppress and cleanse ourselves from feeling "dirty." It was around this time that I revisited my disco experience as a young girl.

Some extreme cases have reported women's oesophagus being irritated and even ruptured, causing blood to come out in their vomit. Some have had blood vessels pop in their eyes because of the violent surge and impact vomiting had on their body.

Trust me, you don't want to do this. I cried out to God for seven years before I was totally free from bulimia. I hated and even abhorred the fact that I was captive to it.

Scotland—The Opportunity of a Lifetime

In the summer of 2002, at the age of 28, I studied spiritual warfare and prayer for three months. This training was offered in an old castle right on the water in West Kilbride on the East coast of Scotland. I fundraised all my tuition and costs and took off on an epic and wild adventure with Jesus. Talk about lush, green intoxicating beauty! Though a little too damp and rainy for my taste, it was an unforgettable experience nonetheless.

I still struggled with bulimia and dealt with a lot of anger on this trip. I believe it was all the anger I had about Ben and my emotional and verbal constipation. I actually kept a journal during that school. Here are a few exerts from it;

June 24, 2002: "I feel like my insides are screaming and closing in on me. Why? What is happening? Such turmoil within me and I'm feeling claustrophobic."

July 24: "How much longer, God, 'til I'm free? You put me together; I didn't ask to be this way! I feel stuck, and You're the only One who can set me free!"

August 17: "I am so angry and fed up! What's blocking me?"

September 15: "God, I want to live and not die. I no longer want to hide behind myself. I feel as though I've been dead so many years, sleeping and not fully awake and alive."

September 25: "How I wish I could cry and let this out. My heart is hurting, pounding, and feels like its bleeding."

Everybody Deserves Joy

Growing up, I never really laughed much. The older I got, the less I seemed to laugh. Over the years I even had people pray for me so that I could laugh again. I found it a little disheartening, because for the longest time when people prayed I would find myself crying instead of laughing.

Eventually, I felt nothing, but at least I no longer cried! I believe it was as though all the "junk" had to be removed from the basement of my heart before it could be replaced with light and joy. But I kept pursuing it until I found it. I was on a mission and didn't give up until I had what I believed was rightfully mine.

It is one of life's greatest gifts, and nothing compares to a good belly laugh! Seriously. If I could only do three things for the rest of my life, I think these would be my choices:

1. Be in nature
2. Worship
3. Laugh

We don't know what we are missing until we are unable to laugh anymore. Nothing releases stress quite like it!

One night during school, my roommate and I were laying in our beds ready to fall asleep. But suddenly without warning, we started laughing. We are talking gut-wrenching belly laughs, the kind where your ribs and stomach cry out for mercy! I don't even know what set us off!

I'm smiling even as a write. That was a monumental day in my life, and I have experienced many of those days since. It felt like something broke inside of me that day, like the floodgates of joy were open and I felt an incredible release! What a gift.

"Come Away with Me," Said My Beloved

I extended my trip by two days after my schooling was done to explore the territory. I figured if I was ever going to live out my "Braveheart" romance with God, Scotland was the perfect setting for it! Laugh all you want—a woman is allowed to dream, right?

I took a ferry to the Island of Arran and I walked on the side of the ocean, watching seals and ocean life doing their thing.

But as per usual, I was drawn to the hills and I could hear them calling me. After a few hours, I ended up at the base of a mountain. I smiled and started trekking in my sandals, jeans, and daypack. For me to worship God in the outdoors was a sure recipe to experience His presence.

The view was spectacular, and it was as if I was following His lead. He was playing with me. He was like an untamed Lover introducing me to a territory I had never explored before. We were young, wild, and free, and I felt giddy. I was being romanced by the King of Heaven. His nearness, His rawness, was tangible. I was scaling the Scottish hills with my fearless Warrior.

When I got to the top, I held off from looking at the view until I inserted my *Braveheart* CD in my portable disc player. If you remember the opening scene from *Braveheart*, the music is playing, and you see the mountains covered with eerie, greyish clouds.

Well, guess what (yes, I know you are rolling your eyes right now): the first song from the movie played as I looked up and around. It was as though I were reliving the movie intro, live in person! I was so touched that I literally fell to the ground and thanked Him for spoiling me. I was humbled that the King of Heaven would know me so intricately and that He would so lavishly grant me the desires of my heart.

It was beautiful, sweet, and romantic. It was true bliss.

No earthly man has ever come close to romancing me like God did that day.

There are plenty more examples of how He spoiled and loved on me so intimately, but those are between us. I am nothing special and far from perfect. This is simply how *awesome* He truly is, and His love is nothing short of extravagant for each and every one of us. This type of relationship or intimacy is available to all who say yes to Him. He is a gentleman who won't force Himself on us. If I asked you to be my friend and you said no, I would not keep pushing. I would respect your choice and decision. God is kind of that way with us.

He already made the first move; it's up to us to respond to Him now. The ball is in our court.

March 17, 2003—A Day to Remember!

A short time after I came back from Scotland, I attended a conference in Edmonton which was about a three-hour drive from Calgary. The conference was great, and the trip there and back was quite eventful. I cried and wailed the entire six-hour drive. At times I felt as though I couldn't breathe—like my chest was closing in on me—but I just kept driving. I wasn't going to get in the way of whatever was taking place. I let it run its course. To most people that would seem like a negative, but considering the outcome, this was an epic day.

Hang with me as I try to articulate my experience. Up until that time I had struggled with hopelessness and suicidal thoughts. To help you understand, here is a glimpse into my heart condition from my journal.

"Why can't I get rid of this death, anger, suicide, and hopelessness? God, I don't feel like You are coming through! I can barely go on another day. Like Jacob, Lord, I'm going to wrestle You, and I'm not going home tonight until I'm free. This is hell, Lord! Your promise of life abundantly ... well, any day now!"

Once I got back from the conference, I parked my car on the edge of a cliff in Calgary. The torment was too real. I felt black clouds physically come out of me. I was as close as ever to actually ending my life that night. I could feel the battle, like I was pinned to the seat. I managed to start the car, but my arms were unable to shift it into gear. I felt like everything in me was screaming "do it" but something was holding back my body from going through with it. It was a similar experience to how I felt back in high school on that dirt road.

Eventually, things settled down, and I felt completely empty as though I had been run over mentally, physically, emotionally, and spiritually. I hung out with God until I was "together" enough to drive back to my apartment.

On that night, my suicidal thoughts, depression, hopelessness, and infatuation with death were defeated. *They died* and not me! My journal entry stated, "Today life and death were set before me, and I chose *life*!"

I've never had a suicidal thought since. *Ever.* Thank you Jesus.

For me, freedom, contentment and peace have *never* been attainable apart from God. The Enemy comes to steal, kill, and destroy, but Christ has come to give us life abundantly! BAM! You have no idea how life-changing and liberating this was.

If you are struggling today with bondage and baggage of any kind, I just want to encourage you to *never* give up. Just because you may not see the sun doesn't mean it isn't shining behind that grey cloud. This too shall pass. Do not lose heart!

Seek help and do not suffer alone. Life is too short to just "exist" and wither away in a slow death. Life *can* be beautiful and worth living and you can have a joyful and peace-filled heart if you do not give up.

As someone who has been there, know that you are not alone, and you are worth fighting for! If I can do it, so can you. Trust me. I had to make the choice to stand back up, to bounce back and to not give in when I got knocked down. So rise from your ashes!

You can do this!

> "Getting knocked down in life is a given. Getting up and moving forward is a choice."
> —Zig Ziglar

CHAPTER 7

"I Do":
In Sickness and in Health

"A perfect marriage is two imperfect people who
refuse to give up on each other."
—Anonymous

I think you understand by now how deeply ingrained my
inability to express myself really was. It was a huge denominator in all of my addictions and issues over the years, and my
marriage was about to suffer because of it as well.

I met Steve in the winter of 2003 through mutual friends
from church. He was from Abbotsford, BC, and was living in
Calgary at the time. He worked for a Christian drug rehab
that he had recently graduated from. We hit it off instantly.
Steve had amazing parents and a solid upbringing and had
recently kicked a nasty heroin addiction he struggled with
throughout his teen years.

He was dark haired, blue eyed, affectionate, gentle, and
had wisdom beyond his years. He was a good honest man and
a true encourager. We had a lot in common, from our faith to
working out and enjoyed the simple things in life. Although

he was not the crying type at all, he was highly sensitive and tender-hearted. But like every couple, we had our differences as well! He was more fearful and laidback while I was the go-getter and fearless adrenaline junky.

Steve continued working at the centre until we got married the following July. I also left my job at the church after four years, and we both worked for a landscaping company. It didn't take long before his fears were exposed but I didn't see how bad it was until we were married. Steve suffered from a serious anxiety disorder and depression.

He would find a job, and soon after start experiencing panic attacks. His fears and insecurities would get the best of him, and he would just drop his things and go home. Over the years, he would leave jobsites, lose his jobs, and get second chances until his bridges were burned. His anxiety was so bad that at times he couldn't even leave our apartment.

His anxiety especially attacked him when he tried anything new, which made it difficult for him to keep a job. He probably spent over half of our seven-year marriage unemployed. He started many goals and dreams but lacked the perseverance and confidence to complete any of them. He sought counselling for years, but nothing seemed to help. It was disheartening and very difficult for me, to say the least. I was the breadwinner and the stable half. Our one-income family made it difficult for us to get ahead and we lived paycheck-to-paycheck.

At first, I was patient and loving, but having given Ben my all, my tolerance level wasn't quite the same with Steve. After addressing the issues at the beginning of our relationship, I quickly noticed just how fragile he was. He had no self-esteem and had a paralysing fear of failure. The minute I tried to gently challenge him, he crumbled.

So I spent the next seven years protecting his heart instead of confronting these issues. He always felt that who he was and what he did were flawed and never good enough. He was shackled and loved the routine of a small sheltered life.

That fall, I started working for a well- known and respected ministry where I spent the next ten years as an employee. I met some incredible folks there and was very blessed to serve alongside them. One of my biggest passions was helping people, and this position gave me the opportunity to do just that.

The first couple of years, I was responsible for answering all the mail, emails, and calls that came into the ministry. These letters could be related to any topic under the sun: marriage, addictions, God, family issues … you name it, and I likely answered it.

About two years into the position, I pioneered and managed a national network of chaplains who provided emotional and spiritual care to victims of crisis and disasters across North America. I grew this nationwide team of responders from one to 250 through crisis training and equipping.

Apart from Steve's lack of employment and struggle with anxiety, we did have a good marriage, and we were both content with each other and life overall.

Steve had his issues, but trust me, so did I.

Insecurity Breeds Jealousy

None of us are perfect, and each partner brings their own baggage. The pain from the damage done by Ben trickled into our marriage. My self-confidence, which had always been an issue, was completely annihilated, and I was insanely jealous and felt threatened the minute a pretty girl walked by. I used to have a pretty sheltered and idealistic worldview, but after Ben I was jaded, and I painted all men with the same brush.

I found myself being the one with serious trust issues which caused me to be controlling and insecure.

I lost it when Steve checked out other women because somehow I felt disqualified from being desirable in his eyes. I was being triggered, and I was reliving my emotions with Ben. It was as if I were taken back eight years and the symptoms were just as intense. I would feel a lump in my throat, become nauseous, cry and shake, and feel stabbed in the heart. In a rage, I snapped and accused Steve of being a flirt or pervert (even though he wasn't).

He was paying for Ben's mistakes.

My self-hatred was through the roof. I started competing and comparing myself to other women, big time. But I only did that when *he* was around, otherwise, I was confident and I didn't care. He also liked skinny girls but dark haired, and now I was blond with an athletic build—not the Skinny Minnie he was into.

Poor Steve! I put him through hell with all that nonsense. He was loving, patient, caring, and so supportive through it all. I could not have asked for a better husband that way.

I know this sounds petty and pathetic! I'm embarrassed to even write this, but these are very real struggles many young *and old* women go through. The only difference is that most of us don't make it public knowledge!

So many of us don't feel pretty enough, blond enough, skinny enough, perky enough. Our tatas and booties aren't big or small enough. And darn it, if there is a flaw to be found we will find it, put it under the magnifying glass, and obsess over it! We are our own strictest judges and absolute worst enemies.

When I was younger, I cared more about having the perfect body and keeping a certain image. Now in my forties, I find myself more comfortable in my own skin, totally accepting, loving and embracing my imperfections and the body my mamma gave me!

Nothing God creates is mediocre and that includes you.

Finding My Voice!

One of the best gifts Steve ever gave me was that he taught me to express myself, be myself, and learn to say no. He had a way of shooting from the hip and pulling off my people pleasing mask. It was a very challenging and uncomfortable process. However, I was so tired of living to prove myself and people please that I didn't care about this foreign discomfort.

I was finally ready to start being "*me.*"

It was a gradual metamorphosis of peeling off the layers of my imposter and becoming authentic and vulnerable. Through trial and error, I quickly realised that people still loved me just the way I was: raw, unpolished, and true. Talk about a refreshing, healing, and freeing revelation!

Even though I still care about what others think about me, I've developed more of a "take me or leave me" attitude. If you like it, stick around, and if not, there's plenty more people out there for you to connect with! I don't click with everyone, and that is OK.

I think we all struggle with fear of man or rejection to a certain extent. And that is why people flock to genuine and real people because it is refreshing and something we all crave deep down. We live in a mean and nasty world, and there aren't too many people out there willing to let it all hang out, humanness and all. We all long for a safe refuge, acceptance and love.

The years passed, and Steve's anxiety and low self-esteem did not improve. He didn't make it easy for me either. He felt threatened by my work, as though I was putting my job before him. One time I stayed a little longer at work because I was counselling a man who was suicidal. We were on the phone for just over two hours. It goes without saying that this was a life-threatening situation.

Even though I was only 15 minutes late, when I finally got to the car, he lost it and gave me heck for putting my job before him. He was always on my case to quit my job so that we could "live on love" and move into our car together. That type of comment and his unhealthy codependence were a real turnoff. That behaviour reminded me of Ben. I gave in to Ben because I was afraid of him, but I wasn't afraid of Steve, so I kept on working and providing for us as a couple.

Steve also battled depression. Every other day I would hear him say "I wish God would just take me." He felt like he had no purpose or value and figured I would be better off without him. To come home or get calls at work from someone so down and tormented all the time was stressful and a heavy burden to carry. I felt like he had no life outside of me, and it was just plain draining.

"Roid" Rage

We were married about one year when we got a gym membership. Being an extremist, all or nothing type of guy, he quickly went knee-deep into the bodybuilding scene. Unfortunately for him, he suffered from the opposite complex that I had (which is so common for men): he could not pack on weight or muscle mass, no matter how hard he tried, and always wished he were bigger.

I, on the other hand, gained muscle mass just thinking about working out.

So, in his true extremist form, he went to steroids to remedy his situation. As if it wasn't enough for me to deal with my monthly three-day PMS nightmare, he now had his own PMS symptoms! If you have ever lived with someone on steroids, you are likely laughing right now as you know what I'm talking about! Now we weren't dealing with depression as much as the rage and emotional instability that accompanied steroid use.

Unfortunately, depending on the type of steroid he used, he saw results. He flipped from steroid to steroid like a fish out of water for a few years. It became his obsession, purpose, and newfound identity. Apart from our faith, working out became our life and our scene. We made a lot of great friends at our gym which was a positive for us. Some of those friendships I still maintain to this day.

We both thought about competing, but knowing our personality types we thought it would be best not to go to that extreme. That lifestyle is all-consuming, and I didn't want to risk an eating disorder resurrecting in me which was all too common in that field.

Bye-bye, Bulimia! Bye-bye, Anorexia!

Two years into our marriage, we both had a desire to move closer to one of our families. Long story short, we ended up moving to Abbotsford where his family lived, and I was able to keep my job and work remotely.

It was at this point that my eating disorders came to a complete halt. Woohoo! Thank you, Jesus!

I was about 31 years old, and I still struggled with my food intake even though I was eating fairly normally. I was maybe 90% free from it, but that nagging ten percent of me controlled *what* I ate. I still entertained the mindset of *allowed* and *not allowed* foods.

Until …

One day, Steve challenged me to start the protein diet for two weeks, and he promised I would not gain weight. I was going to eat five meals a day and not put on weight? Yeah right. But I did it! I hopped on the bandwagon and guess what: I didn't gain any weight. I felt better, had more energy, and maintained my weight even though I was eating more. I was eating "clean." The regimen consisted of meat, nuts, veggies, and fruit, minus carbs, sugar, and processed foods.

Finally, all the years of therapy, prayer, and being tenacious for my freedom finally paid off! That was the cherry on top that set me free. My all or nothing, "good or evil food" mentality was gone. Eating lean meat was actually good to help build muscle, and my preoccupation with food and controlling my portions was over and done with. I am not sure if you realise what a huge breakthrough this was for me!

When the Son sets us free, we are really really free!

I ate like any other normal person, and I continue to do so to this very day. I never think about food unless I need to eat, and eating to me is kind of like putting fuel in my car. If I expect my body to be well and perform at its peak level, I need to give it the nutrients and fuel it needs.

Unlike the day I was delivered from depression and suicide, the eating disorder was a long gruelling process. About six months after I started that protein diet, the lights went on that I was totally and completely free. It was as if the lingering habits just fell off and it was over. I was anorexic from 16–20 and bulimic from 23–30. The battle had finally been won.

Ahhhhhhhh!

If you are struggling today or know someone who is battling this disorder, no matter how severe or mild, you *can* totally be free from it *if* you want. Without it being a debilitating or extreme case, many women have a mild but ever-present struggle and obsession with their weight, and that just plain sucks.

Some women will skip lunch or starve all day if they know they have a special meal that night. They will try to lose weight before going on a trip. Others will binge drink to the point of being sick because they can't handle those calories sitting in them. Meanwhile others will starve or restrict themselves if they had a treat or dessert to cancel out those extra calories.

Sound familiar? You don't need to be stuck in these rituals.

Anything in moderation *is* permissible. Food is not your enemy, and neither is the scale. If it changes your mood from happy to angry, *throw it out!* No inanimate object should have control over you! Replace the numbers on your scale with the following word:

BEAUTIFUL. Because that is what you are.

Fear of Rejection Sabotages Relationships

We had great friends from church and our gym, but Steve had a hard time getting "close" to people. The minute we would start building relationships, he would find a way to ruin them. He would only let people in to a certain point and then push them away. We would go to church but never be able to commit anywhere or get actively involved because every church and person was flawed somehow. He would put an end to promising friendships for no reason and he always had to be right.

It was extremely frustrating. But being the peacekeeper that I was, not wanting to rock the boat, I bit my tongue and just followed along. I personally think he was deeply afraid of rejection. It was as though everyone had to agree with his opinion. Otherwise, he took it personally. It made for an unpleasant social life where I walked on eggshells all the time.

As long as we stayed home and did our own little thing, everything was great. The fact that I couldn't confront Steve on any of his issues was beginning to take a real toll on me. I was getting more and more frustrated, discouraged, and bitter. I was resentful of the fact that I prayed for him so much, and yet God didn't seem to be answering those prayers. His torment was never alleviated.

Steve always wanted me to get a nine-to-five desk job, but that would have been a slow suffocating death for me. My role allowed me to make a difference in people's lives which was my greatest heart's desire. Being able to give of myself by offering hope and comfort to those who had lost so much was very humbling, rewarding, and at times, heartbreaking.

There is no greater honour than to be trusted with someone's wounded heart and innermost pain.

Superficial conversation was uncomfortable for me. However, if you told me that you were abused or suicidal, I would have been right there with you. It is by far easier for me to dive to the depths with someone than to remain on the surface. I felt awkward and like I was wasting my time and theirs. I always admired and envied my brother for his gift of gab and ability to break the ice and strike up conversations with complete strangers. Different strokes for different folks, I guess. That's why we can't compare ourselves with others but thrive in the gifts and abilities we've been given.

The first three disasters I was sent to were Hurricane Katrina and two floods. One was in Terrace, B.C., and the other in Fredericton, N.B. During the ministry's infancy, I was away for long periods of time trying to get this program off the ground. Every time I had to travel for work, it became an increasing stressor on our relationship. His fears and insecurities got the better of him, and he would often quit jobs while I was away, perhaps to prove a point.

However, instead of feeling compassion for his torment, it angered me.

The Downward Spiral Begins

Around 2008, I started feeling a bit tired and overloaded. Out of concern from their observation, a couple of friends warned me that I was headed for burnout. But once the machine is going and you are in the middle of the rat race, how do you pull back? How do you get out?

In 2010 I was expected to send 500 responders to provide emotional and spiritual care to the Vancouver Olympics in the case of a crisis. Needless to say, I didn't quite meet the quota so I felt like a failure right off the bat. I didn't have a support team apart from a few willing volunteer chaplains. The entire year leading up to the Olympics was stressful and exhausting.

During the actual Olympics, I worked 90 hours in overtime alone in one month. But I was the only one to blame as I failed to set boundaries and did not have enough self-care practices in place.

Great things did happen from our presence there, but on a personal level, this deployment was the cherry on top—the one that took the carpet from under me. Nothing traumatic happened, but my body, mind, and heart felt battle-weary.

Without getting into details, my job had its share of challenges, disappointments to swallow, and limited support. At this point, I was also growing in compassion fatigue. Although I did my best to voice my opinions and needs, it often seemed to fall on deaf ears. So my conclusion was just to do my job as best as I could and try not to rock the boat.

Once again, I felt misunderstood and like my voice didn't matter.

Many of the pressures I felt were self-imposed. I expected nothing short of perfection and excellence, both in my integrity and performance. Although unrealistic and exhausting at times, those standards served both as a blessing and a curse. I did what most individuals do on the verge of burnout, and that was to keep going and pretend like everything was OK. In reality, I was about to hit the wall. For me to take a step back would have equalled failure in my own eyes.

But like so many of us *caregivers* and especially "helping professionals," we keep our struggles to ourselves from fear of people thinking we aren't fit for the job or that we can't handle it. We fear being misunderstood and avoid the possible repercussions of being vulnerable about our true condition, so we say nothing.

The result? Burnout and compassion fatigue.

Compound all these things together, once the Olympics were over, and I was exhausted, fed-up, and discouraged. I was always the type of person who valued integrity, honesty, discipline, and doing the right thing no matter what. I was unwavering in my convictions until I hit my wall and my heart got infested with discouragement and disappointment. One of the symptoms of burnout and compassion fatigue is that we lose our ability to care. Not only for others but for ourselves, our lifestyles, and choices. We give up on life in a sense. The following proverb was the truest depiction of my heart condition at the time.

> "Hope deferred makes the heart sick,
> But desire fulfilled is a tree of life."
> —Proverbs 13:12

I had honestly become sick with disappointment.

God wasn't healing Steve, my frustrations at work were not being addressed, and I had a few other personal disappointments with God that were impacting my faith on a subconscious level. I felt like I had nothing left to give. I became infected with hopelessness that nothing was going to improve despite me giving my all. I was now operating in my own strength instead of relying on God's strength to work through me. (Which never works out in the end!)

When we rely on our own strength and our own supply, we always run out! A car cannot operate on empty and neither can we. For me personally, self-care practices work to a certain extent, but when I spend time in God's presence, it is there that I am truly restored and filled up. His well never runs dry. Jesus never experienced burnout, because He operated out of a place of rest and not striving. He was constantly connected to His unlimited supply. Regardless of your faith— as caregivers, I believe there are some real lessons to be learned about His caregiving model.

I guess that deep down, I still felt as though I had something to prove and I was putting myself through the ringer to do so.

My inability to articulate my emotions and condition was about to wreak havoc in my life, yet *again*.

None of us are immune to the steep cost of caring for others. It can cost you your health, your job, your spouse, your family, and it is not worth it. Eventually, our effectiveness as caregivers declines, and we are left walking around disillusioned and apathetic.

In the next chapter, I will share what may be the most difficult part of the book for me to divulge. I am nervous, scared, uneasy, and fearing the worst. I know God has forgiven me, and I have forgiven myself. So I cannot let my fear of your rejection or judgement stop me from sharing my most fragile condition and "ugliness" with you. The only reason I can expose the shameful parts of my story and be *raw* is to help prevent anyone else from making the mistakes I made.

In case you haven't noticed, there are many micro lessons woven throughout my story as to what to do, but also what *not* to do.

We never know the ripple effect that one poor choice will have on our lives until it's too late. There is no better way for me to destroy the "perfect" imposter in me and my debilitating fear of rejection than by letting it all hang out right now.

> "Burnout is what happens when you try to avoid being human for too long."
> —Michael Gungor

CHAPTER 8

'Til Death Do Us Part: Overtaken by Grief

"Love me when I least deserve it, because that is
when I need it most."
—Swedish Proverb

Up until this point, no one knew the challenges we faced in our relationship. I know Steve was happy and on the surface our marriage was fine. However, resentment was building inside me from years of unarticulated frustration with his debilitating anxiety.

I felt more like his mom than his wife. He felt more like my boy than my man.

I couldn't think or focus, and I was exhausted and irritable all the time. I also stopped caring. I gave everything I had during the Olympics and once they were over it felt like, "Now what?" There was no debriefing or discussion about the whole ordeal. It was highly anticlimactic, to say the least.

I wasn't expecting a pat on the back, but any form of acknowledgement for my effort and commitment would have been welcome. Whenever I speak on leadership, I always encourage leaders to affirm the *efforts* of their team as much as their *wins*. Because when we don't win and a project crashes, players lose their sense of worth and feel as though their contributions didn't matter. I can almost guarantee they will not have the same dedication and passion for future projects.

I felt deflated, and life felt flat without the constant push and adrenaline pumping.

The Porn Invasion

It was around this time that Steve's pornography addiction was brought to the light. It was like adding vinegar to *my* already open heart wound in this area. I suspected his issue with porn for years, but he kept denying it until I caught him in the act. It hurt and was very upsetting to me, especially after the sexual trauma I experienced with Ben (which I did not get into in this book as some things are better left unsaid).

Somehow I felt betrayed and my feelings of being inadequate were reinforced in me. I knew it was a coping mechanism for Steve so I refrained from shaming him. I made him promise to at least continue to be open and honest about it. When the urge came on, I told him to come to me instead. It seemed like it helped a bit because I believe that whatever is permissible loses its power and attraction in a sense. We always want what we can't or shouldn't have.

Unfortunately, this was solidifying my view that all men were scum and pigs. I believed that real women would never be enough for men no matter what they looked like. In my wounded and jaded opinion, all men were bound to cheat, watch porn, or go to strip clubs.

The effects of porn on women are much more profound than we would ever care to admit as individuals and society. But don't kid yourselves, the damaging effects impact the viewer just as much as the spouse. I read once that over half of divorce cases reported having pornography as *one* of the major causes for the split.

Some of you may think that I am overreacting since everyone does it and that it's no big deal. However there is more and more research revealing that the effects are highly negative and destructive on so many levels. Just like eating disorders are not simply about a girls' weight, pornography is not just about *getting off.*

Steve was working at this time, and he told me about a girl he was attracted to at his job. He confessed that his thoughts about her were growing more and more but reassured me he wasn't going to act on them. Even though it hurt, at least he was honest enough to admit it to me (something I encourage couples to do *before* they hit the sack with someone, because at that point it's too late). Sure, it may hurt and cause a few fights, but the alternative usually takes couples to the point of no return.

On my end, there was a part of me seeking the next challenge and adventure. First of all, that was my personality type, and secondly, life had not been normal for the past few months. All of a sudden, the routine felt uncomfortable. Steve kept pushing me to go on a week holiday to Mexico, but it wasn't my thing. Renting a cabin in the bush or going on a wild outdoor adventure would have been more my beat. To this day, I still regret not listening to my inner voice and practising self-care the way I knew worked for me.

The stars were aligning for disaster on both ends. Temptations were meticulously orchestrated to trip us up. We weren't going to church much at this point because Steve was unhappy everywhere he went. That was mistake number one for us. We focused on outward stimuli to fulfil what we knew only God could.

Long story short, I gave in and went to Mexico for a week, *by myself*. Big mistake. I was bored all week. I was lonely, I danced, played volleyball, took boxing lessons, and read by the pool. Who goes South by themselves anyways? I went because the trip was free with my travel points. The cabin, on the other hand, would have cost us money we didn't have. To be frugal and wise, I figured my hubby knew best.

> "I don't have nothing to regret at all in the past, except that I might've unintentionally hurt somebody else."
> —Jimi Hendrix

My Trip South Went South

Like most people who go to resorts, I had a few drinks here and there. One night, I had more than a few. To be honest, I was intoxicated and I screwed up big time. I don't even remember much about that night, let alone the guy's name, but I had a one night stand. It is perhaps the biggest and most haunting regret of my life. How I wish I could rewind time. The regret of my subsequent actions ate away at me for years to come, and it still does.

What I do know is that one mistake—one bad choice— changed my life and my marriage forever.

It was *the seed* that grew into a nightmare of events to follow.

I was in the wrong 100%. There is no denying that. I have had to live with the consequence of my actions, and the guilt and shame that came with them. I have a list of reasons

I could share to help justify my actions, but I have zero intention of even going there because only cowards do that. What is done is done, and I own up to my mistakes.

However, there is one factor I wish to explore with the hope that others can learn from my experience.

I desperately wanted things to change for Steve and me, and I wanted our marriage to be normal and healthy. But on certain levels, Steve wasn't healthy. I wanted to tell him to grow up, be a man, hold a job, but I could never tell him that to his face. I wanted things to be different, and subconsciously I believe that this was my way of forcing change.

I was unable to express my needs, desires, or frustrations. I was pent up, and I acted out. As in my past, it was my way of saying, "Everything is NOT fine."

It is critical that we always keep open communication even if we think it will hurt our spouse. If we skirt around issues to *protect* their little hearts, it will just come back to bite us later. Trust me. Maybe it's a temptation, an addiction, your frustrations in the marriage, or your lack of fulfilment. I don't care what your problem is—we all need to man up and tell it like it is. Like the famous line from *A Few Good Men*, "You can't handle the truth." You better learn to handle it. Otherwise, that truth will cost you.

The other thing I want to mention about communication is if you aren't having fulfilling conversations, one of you is likely going to look for that connection elsewhere! The stimulating conversations with the plumber or the secretary will all of a sudden make them look like a heartthrob. Especially if one mate is on the road a lot or emotionally unavailable, temptation can arise on either side.

Plus, we cannot belittle the power of our words. It is imperative that we build each other up and show appreciation for one another. Go ahead, make your spouse feel wanted, desired, loved, and beautiful.

Because let me tell you: if *you* don't somebody else will.

If you are having an emotional affair or entertaining the thought of going through with a sexual one, I cannot urge you enough *not* to. Talk openly and frankly with your spouse about your unmet needs and desires. The grass is *never* greener on the other side, and it likely won't change anything. Communication is always key. If you think your marriage sucks now, multiply your situation times ten. Infidelity is never an option, a solution, or a way out.

The Evil One comes to steal, kill, and destroy, and there is nothing he loves more than to destroy marriages. It deeply impacts the kids, affects your job and health, brings despair and confusion, and affects all areas of life. Whether you believe in God or the Devil is irrelevant. But you will likely agree that the family unit is not what it used to be, and as a result, society is suffering and reaping the consequences.

It all starts in the home.

I remember lying in bed that night at the resort, seeing my wedding ceremony playing out in my head. The whole week after I got back, I couldn't eat or sleep, and I was nauseous to the point of puking. And I'm not talking self-induced. It was the worst feeling in the world, and I ended up telling Steve the whole truth about that night.

I was afraid he might react violently, but he stayed calm. I think he was in shock. Steve trusted me completely. I had only slept with Ben previous to him, so this was totally out of character for me to act out this way.

But my story is a real life example of the cost of burnout/compassion fatigue when left unattended. You don't care about your actions or their consequences. Moral decay is one of the costliest symptoms. We all have the capacity to go there; I don't care who you are.

You do things that are completely out of character because you can't afford to care. When you layer disappointment on top of disappointment, eventually caring is too costly. At least if we stop "expecting" good then we aren't so deflated when good things don't happen.

We are human first and foremost. Never forget that. None of us are above anyone else or any "sin."

We *all* have a breaking point.

Steve was deeply hurt, and with reason. He didn't know how to handle it. The more time went by, the more unstable he became. He made me confess to our friends and family, which I believe was partially a form of payback to humiliate me.

Around that same time, my grandmother passed away. Grandma was 101 years old and a woman I truly loved and admired. She had become one of my best friends over the years, and saying goodbye was not an option for me. I went to Ontario for the funeral, but Steve didn't want me to go because he felt I was putting my family before him. During the five days I was gone, he quit his job and blamed it on me.

The interrogation on Steve's part was relentless. I tried to deal with it as best I could, but nothing worked. His parents were obviously upset that I had hurt their boy. We had a bit of a family meltdown, and we didn't see his parents for over a month.

We found ourselves *alone.* Nothing good comes out of isolation, even if you are an isolated couple.

Slow Road to Destruction

At this point, Steve had alienated us from our church friends, so we were on our own spiritually. Nothing seemed to help him get "unstuck" from the wound. So we decided that maybe the best thing for us would be to have fun together. We started going out for dinner and drinks. What started out as occasional outings became weekly rituals.

Someone very close to Steve had just gone through a nasty divorce and was going down a similar road that we were on. The only problem was that he was one step ahead of us. Like any other addictive personality, the gradual progression of highs needed to increase. Drinking was apparently not cuttin' it.

Our desire and intentions were good, but the means of getting there was all wrong.

So we tried a couple of "soft" drugs, as we were willing to do anything to help us rekindle our love for one another. But we were in a real tug of war because we felt convicted and "dirty" after doing them. We would be "good" for a while but then think, "Who cares?" and end up going there again.

Obviously, nothing worked. We were having some fun together but deep down we knew it wasn't right. We didn't know what else to do or who to go to for help. This lifestyle is all fun and games for a while, but in the end it always leads to destruction. You can't play on the Devil's playground and leave unscathed. He doesn't play fair and takes no prisoners!

My New Little Friend

One night, I was introduced to a white powdery substance that would become my new "little friend." Of all the drugs in this world, it was the only one I had ever been intrigued by or curious about. I had never tried cocaine, but from what Ben had told me it sounded like my kind of high. The seed that was planted 15 years earlier was now about to germinate.

After being down and depressed most of my life, I was not into downer drugs but attracted to the *picker upper* effects of cocaine. Steve kept encouraging me to try it that night, and I honestly don't think I ever would have done it had he not been there cheering me on. I was totally scared since I didn't know what to do or what to expect. Finally, I gave in, which again wasn't like me. I knew it was wrong, but I didn't care.

So up it went, my first line of cocaine. I didn't know that this little friend would almost cost me my life.

When I say "my little friend," nothing could be further from the truth. Cocaine will strip you of all common sense and empty your bank account. It will make you do things you never dreamed you were capable of doing. It will steal your moral compass and potentially kill you. It will never satisfy but rather leave you desperate and risking your life for more. Cocaine hijacks your brain and eventually makes you believe you can't live without it.

If you are entertaining the thought of using any drug, I cannot caution you enough *not* to go there. Obviously, not everyone who experiments with drugs becomes an addict, but we never know if we will unless we try. So it is best we do not give it the opportunity to sink its teeth into us. The fact that we can become prisoners of synthetic chemicals infuriates me!

My personal belief is that God is the ultimate high we can experience in this world. His presence is like a drug, as it satisfies but always leaves you wanting more, in a good way! His Enemy cannot create, so he spends his time coming up with counterfeit drugs and things to replace what God created for our good in the first place. As long as we go to anything *but*

God to fill our souls and meet our deepest needs, the Devil is happy and has done his job. By God's grace, I hope I never give him that satisfaction again.

Life is too short to live under the dictatorship and at the mercy of substances!

I was often told that the first line was the best and that you would forever chase that same high. That wasn't the case for me. The first was OK, but I couldn't really tell the difference. I didn't *feel* high or anything. All I knew was that I had energy, was talkative, and danced a lot in the living room. That was it for that night.

We promised each other that we wouldn't touch coke again. We looked at it as a one-time deal to appease my curiosity. As much as we wanted to stop this lifestyle, it was as if we couldn't. We were sucked in, and it felt too easy to stay in. Turning away from it meant we had to face our internal realities as individuals and as a couple. And that was not going to happen. Much too painful of a thought—so let's just keep ignoring it and numbing our pain. The next weekend Steve did it with me, but we didn't even drink. We did the cocaine because it put us in a good mood, removed our insecurities, and made us chatter bugs. We were no longer shy or reserved, but able to engage the world around us much more freely.

Since I was in turmoil inside, it didn't take long for me to unknowingly get hooked. I would do a line before I went for my daily walk or workout. It helped me focus, gave me the energy to clean the house, and was the "oomph" to get through my day. It got rid of my tiredness and brain fog which were debilitating at the time. Remember, I was experiencing burnout and compassion fatigue. Cocaine was the perfect remedy to counter my symptoms and make me functional again (at least while the effects lasted).

Instead of using prescription drugs or healthy self-care practices, like many other hurting individuals I chose a destructive coping mechanism. Unfortunately, I didn't feel like I could talk to anyone about it. Drugs were inappropriate and highly taboo, especially in the Christian world. So I began to isolate and turn to my "little friend" because it never judged me. Whenever the pain became unbearable and I needed an escape or picker upper, it was there for me.

Unfortunately, many people have misconceptions about drugs, assuming that all users are strung out and shooting up in dark alleys. They assume dealers all have missing teeth and tattoos from head to toe. Nothing could be farther from the truth. Many users are doctors, lawyers and successful businessmen and drugs don't care what you do for a living, what color your skin is or how much money you have in the bank. If you are human, you have the potential to falling prey to its seducing power. We happen to be talking about drugs right now, but maybe your struggle is shopping, sex, drinking, gossiping, cleaning or gambling. One coping mechanism is not better than another. They are all different but the same.

My struggle never became a daily habit, but more of a mental obsession and craving. Instead of thinking about food 24/7, like in previous years, I was thinking about my little friend and how happy it would make me when we would finally reunite again.

The Beginning of the End

It was all fun and games until one day. Steve walked in the door, and his eyes were different. His pupils were super constricted, and his countenance was "off." I knew then and there: he had just done heroin. I immediately told him, "This is the beginning of the end for you." He said, "Oh no, I'm fine. I have this under control. It was only one time, and I won't do it again," mumbling those words as he nodded in and out of consciousness.

I hated seeing him under heroin's spell. It gave me the heebie-jeebies for some reason.

His anxiety made him long for the peace and wellbeing that heroin falsely provided, and from that point on it was the only drug he touched.

Steve's "partner in use" lived across the parking lot from us, and out of desperation, I thought that moving across the city might make it more difficult for them to hook up. Now I laugh at my naïveté! Drug addiction knows no distance or boundaries and is no respecter of persons.

Steve became more unstable and unrecognisable. One night, he grabbed hold of the steering wheel and swerved us off the road so that we could crash and die together. He went on to take a whole bunch of pills just to end up in the hospital later that same night. Around 4:00 a.m., he ripped off all the intravenous tubes and busted out of that hospital in a tantrum looking to score again. He was very hostile, aggressive, and like a ticking time bomb. It was creepy and unnerving. He was night-and-day different from the Steve I had once fallen in love with.

My Best Friend, My Mentor, My Saving Grace

One night, I went for dinner with a friend of mine who was a mentor and counsellor to me. We had met years before through our church and always kept in touch. We could always dive into deep and real conversations without having to cut through any superficial fluff. It was awesome and refreshing.

This chick was also very in tune with God and had a way of knowing things. She was a woman who was truly crowned with wisdom and compassion. Some of you may understand the term "psychic" or prophetic in Christian terms, but this girl heard from God, which was one quality that made her so incredibly effective in her counselling.

That particular night, we met for dinner at East Side Mario's. I even remember the booth we were in. Right in the middle of dinner, she stopped and said,

"Mel, what are you doing? Are you using cocaine?"

Our relationship changed forever, and over time we became the best of friends. To this day she remains my confidant and counsellor, and I can't imagine where I would be without her voice and presence in my life. Even though we are thousands of miles apart physically, I feel closer to her than anyone else in my life apart from my husband. We "get" each other, and not a day goes by where we don't call, text, or email. She is my accountability partner, and I love her more than words can express.

I want to quickly refer to a story you may have heard about: the story of David and Bathsheba.

King David was a great warrior and leader, but he slept with the wife of one of his most loyal soldiers. To make matters worse, he had her husband killed in battle shortly after the affair. Not long after these events, the prophet Nathan confronted David, and David didn't deny or backpedal in any way. He took full responsibility and ownership for his mistakes.

He knew nothing was hidden from God, and I guess that is the way I felt and still feel. I didn't deny it for a second. My best friend was like my Nathan at that point. When we admit and confess our sins, it gives God room and permission to work in our lives.

I think God revealed it to her because He knew He could trust her with me. He also knew the potential depth of relationship we were about to embark on. After that night, I no longer felt "alone," but I had a trusted friend with whom I could confide in. What a life saver that was and is to this day.

Disturbing Threats

Around mid-July, a couple of weeks after Steve started using heroin, we had a conversation that was a little concerning. He was not in a good space. We were in our apartment, and he was "off." He threatened to kill himself and to kill me if I left him. His thoughts were very dark and all over the place. So I talked to his parents, and they decided to call the police since we didn't know what else to do. Plus, Steve was an obvious danger to us both.

I gave my report, and a restraining order was issued. Sometimes Steve would wait for me at the gym parking lot just to see me. I saw him three times during our one-month separation. He had changed so much that my love for him was growing cold. I felt sorry for him since he looked like a wounded little boy. He started smoking again, was super anxious, and was looking very scrawny. I seriously questioned if it was even possible for us to recover from all of this.

When the restraining order was issued, Steve moved back to his parents' place. I was fearful he might break into our apartment to supply his habit, so I moved everything out of there except for my work and a sleeping bag. I had a friend help me move the couch out of the apartment, but I did the rest all by myself. It was exhausting, and I think my rage and frustration were the fuel and strength I needed to get the job done. From the third story apartment to the U-Haul and from the U-Haul to storage. What a day. Once again, "my little friend" gave me the energy I needed to complete this nearly impossible task.

Dazed and Confused

That was one of the worst months of my life. Anyone who has ever been separated from their spouse knows that separation is painful even when welcomed. I felt so grieved inside, so empty, lost, and confused. I would occasionally read my Bible or worship, but I kept God at a comfortable distance since I knew He would make me walk through the pain and confront it, unlike cocaine which helped me avoid and numb it.

Have you ever hurt so deeply that you were ready to do *anything* to stop the pain?

So I continued to self-medicate with cocaine, especially when I was alone. The ritual in itself was comforting and became my "companion" in my isolation, loneliness, and despair. It seemed to calm the tremor and unsettledness of my soul.

This was one of my lowest points. Even though I had friends, I didn't want to be a needy pest, so I kept to myself a lot of the time. It felt like I was an alien here on earth. It felt like a bad dream from which I couldn't wake up and I cried a bucket of tears. I feared our marriage was over and there was no hope left. The damage had been done. I no longer knew my husband nor did I want anything to do with the man he was becoming.

It has been a very difficult process of loving, accepting, and forgiving myself for the one-night stand. I don't think anything could have be more out of character for me, but if God had forgiven me, I needed to accept His forgiveness and in turn forgive myself. As much as I would love to rewind the tape and undo what was done, I can't. Steve Maraboli said it well:

> "You are not your mistakes, you are not your struggles, and you are here *now* with the power to shape your day and your future."

Alone

Being alone as much as I was gave me a lot of time for self-reflection. I remember observing people while having lunch at a restaurant. I saw parents with their kids, old and young couples, and felt like I wanted to tell them not to take this time for granted. I wanted to tell couples that if they were having issues to work through them because jumping ship wasn't always the answer.

I felt like I wanted to shout from the rooftops, "*Hey*, here is what NOT to do!" Again a major motivator for me to write this book. We never know how much human interaction brings meaning and value to our lives until we are stripped of it and find ourselves alone. None of us were created to be alone, and when we are, it is a dark and restless place to be.

I kept working and tried to maintain my routine as much as possible. I felt so incredibly empty and alone, but that was my own fault. If you know people who are alone without family, don't be afraid to reach out. Just the fact that you make them feel like you "see them" may be all the hope they need to feel special and make their heart smile. Every life matters and every human being has worth.

To be lonely is one of the most profoundly painful feelings a human being can experience. The remedy is not the quantity but the *quality* of relationships. You can be in a crowd of people and still feel completely alone and empty, and on the flip side you can find one friend who *gets* you and feel a deep sense of belonging.

"The most terrible poverty is loneliness and
the feeling of being unloved."
—Mother Theresa

Even in my lowest pit and darkest moment, I knew God was with me. It was a truth I never doubted for a second because I truly believed that nothing could ever separate me from His love.

I was so tired and battle-weary that the thought of having to walk through the grief and pain was unbearable. I couldn't fight anymore. My shame, fears, and addiction kept me from going to Him and instead had me reaching out to my "little friend."

I was so disappointed in myself and was plagued with the thought of having disappointed God.

Every once in a while, God would show up, make Himself known to me, and shower me with His love. I think He was attempting to melt down my barriers and fears despite my attempts to protect myself from my own pain.

One reason for keeping my distance was my lack of trust in life and in God. Have you ever experienced so many disappointments that you became distrustful, fearing the worst and waiting for the next curveball to hit? I had a hard time trusting that life wouldn't rip me off again. Today my life is incredibly beautiful, and fulfilling, yet I still find myself bracing for the next hit, or for the ball to drop. I have to consciously stop myself from entertaining that fear.

It honestly took me about three years before my relationship with God was fully restored and where I could trust Him wholeheartedly again. He never changed—*I did*. I find it interesting how we can see God as all good and all loving as long as our life is good. What happens when we experience a crisis and all of a sudden we don't have all the answers? Here are a few words I believe to be true:

If God was good before the incident or loss, He is still good during and after. What has changed is our perception and attitude because of the assault our hearts have endured. I never stopped loving, fearing or believing in God, but my struggle was in trusting Him.

Funny how people don't believe in God until poop hits the fan and all of a sudden it's His fault!

When a crisis takes place, it makes an imprint on our life and leaves an evident pre and post crisis mark on us. Life as we knew it before the crisis may never be the same and we may permanently be changed as well. One thing I have discovered over and over is that God is good.

He loves to make all things *beautiful.*

Looking back, I can see how losing my job at the time would have potentially been the nail in the coffin for me. It was the reason I got up in the morning and was a stabilising anchor for me at the time. It was like a point of reference for me while everything else was out of order.

Friday 13, August 2010

It was on this night that Steve did heroin for the last time. He was living with his parents, so I did not see him, but he went home around 11:00 p.m. and went straight to bed. Apparently, Steve's parents heard a strange noise coming from the basement between 2:00 and 3:00 a.m., but they assumed it was an animal outside. They went back to sleep.

Unfortunately, it was then that Steve took his final breath.

Around noon the next day, one of Steve's brothers called. I hadn't spoken to him in months, so I did not answer.

My heart is beating out of my chest right now even as I write.

His voicemail message said, "Mel, Steve died last night. Call me."

My heart sank.

I called him back immediately. My first words to him were, "Is this a joke?" He got quite upset at me for thinking it was a joke, but I was obviously in shock. I was alone in my apartment. My legs gave from under me, and I collapsed to the floor. I was dry heaving, dizzy; my body felt tingly, and the room was spinning.

You may as well have punched me in the heart with a cement slab.

Steve's parents thought it would be best if I didn't come home to see Steve. Perhaps they were angry; perhaps they didn't want me to remember him that way. Regardless, I didn't push to see him.

My parents were fully aware of everything we were going through. They flew out for a week to be the awesome parents and friends that they were. Their simple presence and having them by my side was incredibly helpful and comforting, and it also meant I didn't have to go home to an empty apartment. What could have been an unbearable week became somewhat manageable because I had my two pillars by my side. They didn't try to console me or give me false comfort; they simply loved me in my brokenness and my mess.

Although Steve battled heroin addiction during high school, he had been clean for nine years. Just a one-month relapse was all it took to cut his life short. We always think it won't happen to us until it does, and usually it's like a thief in the night.

That could have been me, or any one of us who has ever done drugs. We never know what we are putting in our bodies, and we never know when that one hit will be the kicker. There is a reason we don't see drugs addicts in their 50s and 70s—people who don't quit either end up in jail, the hospital, or the grave.

Even though I shared our weaknesses towards the end, I choose to remember Steve for the man he was for the majority of our time together. I celebrate his strengths and qualities, and I am forever grateful for all the good and the many blessings he brought to my life.

Rest in peace, dear Steve.

When we don't deal with our pain properly, it never ends well. Some people chose more "acceptable" and lower risk coping mechanisms while others go to more extreme means. But we are all human, and we must be quick to love and slow to judge.

It is so easy to judge others when we don't understand what they are going through! We judge when we don't love or when we want to make ourselves feel better about our own inadequacies. We judge others because of our ignorance and lack of understanding of what they are going through.

I don't care what colour, faith, or nationality you are or how much money you have in the bank—the bottom line is that we are *all* human. The more we suffer, the more compassion, love, and understanding we should have for others.

No matter what assaults our hearts endure, the only way to get over pain is through it. No shortcut or avoidance will ever work. We will only find ourselves one or ten years later having to face the same pain.

One reason why God tells us to stay away from certain things is because He knows that in the end, it will only lead to our destruction. He is a loving Father, and just like we warn our kids not to touch a hot stove, He does the same with us because He loves us.

One bad decision only breeds other bad decisions. Eventually, we are so far off track that we don't even recognise the road we are on. The destination ends up being night-and-day different from where our journey was supposed to take us.

We get lost one bad turn at a time.

If you find yourself lost today and using coping mechanisms that you know are hurting you or your family, life is way too short to keep wasting time avoiding the aches of our hearts. You will *not* be able to do this on your own. You will need help from your friends, family, and spouse to walk through this with you.

Stop protecting your spouse from the truth. It's time we all grow thicker skin and face the music. Otherwise, the silence, lies, and denial will only keep us bound and create greater despair. I read once in my favourite book that if we confess our faults to one another, we will be healed.

This is a most liberating truth in my own life.

"He heals the broken-hearted and binds up their wounds."
—Psalm 147:3

CHAPTER 9

The Collapse: My Road to Recovery

> "The things we do to avoid the ache are always worse in
> the end than the ache itself."
> —John Eldredge

The intermission between Chapters 8 and 9 was an interesting one. I felt my chest tightening. I had a hard time breathing, and I just wanted to crawl into a ball, cry, and go to sleep. So I did the opposite. I told my best friend what was surfacing as I wrote, and went for a walk instead.

It worked. My best friend's response was that I was being released from the shame of the affair. She said, "Surgery may be over, but the healing can be uncomfortable." She hit the nail on the head for sure.

In the past, self-condemnation from the affair would have eaten me alive. I was so insanely hard on myself and perfection was the only acceptable goal. I was a martyr who felt the need to whip and punish myself to pay for my mistakes. Obviously, that never worked.

That would have meant that my freedom was the result of my performance and works rather than what Jesus did for me. I have never been able to forgive myself or feel cleansed for my mistakes outside of God. I have been forgiven and therefore I no longer entertain the onslaught of lies that the Enemy occasionally tries to throw at me.

About three weeks after Steve's passing, I moved back home to Ontario. I was unsure how long I would be there, but I had no intentions of staying there long term. I never really liked my hometown, so for me to move back after living in Western Canada for 16 years was traumatic in itself. I didn't want to stay in Abbotsford because everything was a trigger and a reminder of Steve, plus there was nothing there for me. My brother and his wife were beyond generous to have me stay in their loft. I was very humbled and touched by their kindness and hospitality.

Thanks to Steve, who had really pushed me to express myself and remove the masks, my relationship with my parents grew leaps and bounds over the years. God did some amazing work between us, and I was very comfortable sharing my struggles with them at this point. They were an amazing support system for me, and I don't know what I would have done without them.

I thought that moving across the country would be enough for me to leave my "little friend" behind. The cravings and obsession haunted me. I used to go to food to cope with life, but there was no way I was going back to that hell, and although food would have been more "acceptable" to some, in the end, it's all the same.

Not only was I scrambling to kick this addiction, but also Steve's passing created in me a troubled and broken heart. If I could have seen my emotional heart, I believe it would have been bleeding and full of arrows. The grief was unbearable, unsettling, and it was as though I couldn't turn off the turmoil inside. Peace was a distant memory that seemed out of reach. One minute I felt numb and the next I was overtaken by a tsunami of tears. I was dealing with PTSD, complex grief, addiction, my unresolved burnout, and compassion fatigue on top of the cross-country move back home.

You could say I had a full plate of emotions to process.

Vicious Anxiety Attacks

For the first time in my life, I started experiencing panic attacks. I felt rattled, restless, and had destabilising symptoms firing on all cylinders. My world had turned upside down, and it took everything in me not to drink during the week. I would count down the days until Friday when I felt it was acceptable to have a drink. I would drink alone most of the time as an attempt to drown my sorrows and numb the ever-present agitation within my soul.

A few weeks after settling in, I approached an old school friend who I thought may have "connections" to illegal substances. Little did I know, everyone in that scene that I knew had gotten clean in recent years. They thought it was funny, but it sure wasn't funny to me at the time! This old friend from school ended up being my lifeline throughout the next nine months—my confidant and a true lifesaver at the time.

My inward agitation became the catalyst for my reckless quest for cocaine. I went to the city to score and met a biker I thought "looked the part." He was a super nice guy and we hit it off instantly, but he was leery because he had been busted by an undercover cop in the past. For some reason, everyone in that scene thought I was a cop which made it near impossible for me to ever score. Apparently, I didn't look the part since I was too clean looking and seemed like a good person. At least that's what I was told.

So, instead, he told me about a couple spots where I could likely find some. After trying a few places, I came out of there empty handed, but I was determined to score at any cost. I had to stop the turbulence within my heart. This stubbornness and tenacity had served me well in the past but now weren't such a good thing.

I put myself in two very sketchy and life-threatening scenarios, so biker dude finally put me in contact with someone he knew as an attempt to keep me out of harm's way.

I can't say that every high was delightful because it was far from it. There were too many nights when I lay in bed asking God to forgive me and spare my life because I didn't want to die. I felt like I was going to have a heart attack or have my head explode. I promised myself I would never do it again until I could not contain the stirring within.

It was a love-hate relationship with this drug, a real tug of war. It's a mental addiction because it stops your body from releasing its natural production of dopamine. So you always need more coke to balance your levels just to feel normal or good again. Otherwise, you become extremely depressed and the longing to feel "good or happy" again becomes all consuming. Who wants to be down when you know you could be up?

I couldn't be with others, but I also couldn't be by myself. I find this quote to be so very true:

> "Pain is no evil unless it conquers us."
> —Charles Kingsley

When we don't deal with our pain, it will conquer us, plain and simple. I lived for the high and the danger because I was addicted to the adrenaline-filled life. For me to crash and just "be" was highly uncomfortable. I think first responders can relate. You get home from work and life is routine, flat, and boring. So you either go brain-dead watching TV with your six-pack, or you long to go back to work. Others opt for the high-risk reckless behaviours like sex, drugs, gambling, reckless driving, and drinking, just to cope with their hidden PTSD and symptoms of vicarious trauma.

There has been an alarming increase in first responder suicides, and I believe a huge factor is that frontline workers are not able to talk. They suffer alone, and they suffer quietly. Unfortunately, the result can cost a responder and caregiver their life.

About eight months after Steve's death my mentor/best friend had a group of people pray for me. Until that day, I heard tormenting whispers saying, "Steve is in the grave because of you." I believed Steve's death was my fault, and that I had to pay for it. I was freed from that shame and tormenting guilt that night. Those thoughts still occasionally enter my mind, but I just tell them where to go.

February 2011—I Hit My Wall

I was at our office headquarters and had been there a couple of days. I had panic attacks while on the job, so one of my colleagues took me to the hospital. When I got back, I finally told my boss that I needed to take a break. I had hit my wall and knew I could no longer keep going. I took four month's short-term disability from March until June.

On March 1, 2011, I checked myself into rehab. My motivation was not because I thought I had a problem with cocaine, but just to escape *everyone*. I wasn't there to quit as much as I was there to get away, *avoid* all pain and disappear from civilization for a while. Funny enough, my first day there I sat beside a guy who was a heroin addict, and his name was Steve.

Needless to say, it was a long month. I met pretty interesting characters, some of whom I am still in touch with today. The people there were hilarious, and I think that being able to laugh as much as we did was healing in itself.

About halfway through the program, my counsellor sat me down in her office. She was not impressed with me. Apparently, it was obvious that I wasn't taking the program seriously, and she felt I was wasting time and confronted me on it. Little did I know this session would be a life changer for me.

I could never have orchestrated what was about to happen.

I don't remember how I got started on it, but for the next 90 minutes, I felt as though I went into a time warp back to Ben. I was reliving all the major situations of abuse and torture as well as his daily mistreatment and disrespect for me as a human being.

It was the first time *ever* that I was in touch with my anger towards Ben.

I vented as though I were actually speaking to him, standing up for myself and articulating my feelings. I was furious, crying, shaking, and all this pent-up rage I carried for 15 years was finally coming out. You can imagine the release I felt. It was more than welcome and highly overdue!

That was a monumental day in my life. To have a safe place where I could re-enter that relationship and experience the emotions I had denied myself and numbed, and then to release them, was very therapeutic and healing for me—nothing that could have been planned or rehearsed by any means.

I went on to complete my 28 days and have been clean ever since. Now, because of the way cocaine works in the brain, it does not mean I didn't crave it daily for many months to come. Upon my return, I moved in with my parents, which was a harsh blow to my pride. I was a 36-year-old widow moving into my parent's basement after coming out of rehab.

Not the script I would have ever written for myself.

Thank God for my friends and family. I would never have made it without them. That season I felt ashamed, disappointed in myself, and just struggled with the narrative that had become my life.

I was broken, humbled, and RAW.

The Power of a Parent's Love

My friendship with my parents, took a profound turn for the better. I remember that their love, support, and patience were heartbreaking in a good way. I had never gone to them before in crisis because my misconceptions about them had built a wall between us. I had thought their love was dependent on my perfect behaviour. I couldn't be any less perfect at that point, and they embraced me with open arms.

I believe a huge part of my healing was due to them. I was finally able to receive their love fully. The threat of being myself was now gone, and I was safe to be imperfect, flawed, and authentic. It was as if my imperfections, mistakes, and failures were all exposed and out there for judgment, ridicule, and condemnation—instead, I ran into the most powerful force in the world: love. A love revealed through my parents like no other love I had ever known. God used them mightily to bring healing and restoration to my life and heart. I was loved, embraced, and accepted just as I was, and *that* was a game changer for me.

Over the years, I've come to realise that my parents' unconditional love was the key that broke open my heart to trust God again. I can't explain how it happened, but it did. God used them to draw me back to Himself.

God's redeeming love! There is nothing more compelling in this world.

I also want to add that Steve's parents played a significant role in my healing as well. I am sure they had their issues to work through, but they never communicated anything short of God's unconditional love toward me. Their friendship and support over the years have affected me profoundly. We remain great friends, and I love and respect them more than words can say.

Nothing heals like love. Nothing.

The next three months I was on my disability were just plain unpleasant. I struggled with cravings and a lot of unrest within my heart because I was no longer numbing my emotions. For the first time in years, I articulated my sadness, grief, pain, and frustration. I didn't care how it came out; the fact that it came out was good enough for me. I remember thinking I wished I could have learned to express myself years earlier. Can you imagine the hardships I would have avoided?

I was so grateful for the amazing friends who loved and supported me through that time. You know who you are! Slowly but surely, I got better. I was spending more time with God and was committed to moving on and being whole.

My Two Cents

If you know anyone who struggles with any kind of addiction, I encourage you to be there for them. Be patient, listen, and don't pretend to have all the answers because you don't. Most importantly, love them unconditionally, because addicts are known to be highly sensitive individuals.

Shame and fear of rejection often push people back into the safety of their addiction because they know it will never judge or reject them.

Many studies are starting to show that one of the most important factors in someone's recovery is love and *community*. I couldn't agree more because it was in my isolation and my inability to express myself that things progressively got worse for me. However, with true friends, my family support, and counselling, I managed to stay clean.

If anyone tries to get clean on their own without support and community, they likely won't make it. We were made for relationship. Remember the name I gave my drug? It was "my little friend." If no one else came to fill the void after I broke off the relationship with coke, I guarantee I would have fallen back into its arms in no time.

I was starting to feel "normal" again, one year later! But nothing comes easy in life and freedom does not come without a cost. There is a price to pay if we are going to *own* our freedom. I felt as though I was just coming out from the relentlessly overwhelming waters of grief. My head was finally above water.

My peace was restored. I could breathe and be *with* myself again. Life had new colour, the clouds had passed, and I could feel the warmth of the sun beginning to shine on me. I was ready to live again, to laugh again, and to love again. The first week of July I was scheduled to go back to work, and I did.

I was ready to turn the page and put the past behind me.

"Bravery is willingness to show emotional need."
—Richard Gere

CHAPTER 10

Ding, Ding: In the Ring with Cancer

"Every champion was once a contender
that refused to give up."
—Rocky Balboa

I was 36 years old. I walked into my doctor's office for an annual check-up, and he did a breast exam *just in case*. I don't think most doctors do breast exams for women in their mid-thirties so I looked at it as him being thorough and exceptional in care. He felt a small lump but assured me it was likely just muscle tissue.

A biopsy was scheduled, and let me tell you—the pain of having that long needle scrape the inside of my breast was excruciating. The doctor and nurse looked at the screen, and I knew right away by their facial reaction that it was cancer. They had poker faces, but I still knew it. When our time was done, he told me to get my mammogram done right away so that I could kill two birds with one stone. That was further confirmation to me that something wasn't right.

The day after I returned to work, my family doctor called me back in his office. With tears in his eyes, he told me that I had breast cancer. I was in shock. I shed a tear, and when I got to my car I broke down. I sat there weeping as I realised I was knocked down yet again by this unfair script called life. I was in shock and denial. After everything I've just been through—are you kidding me?

I just finished mopping myself off the floor, and now this?

I was still rather fragile from the previous years, and now I had to face this giant? I remember the day all too well. I was in my room in my parent's basement. I had it out with God and made a deal with Him. I told Him, "If anything else is supposed to happen to me this year or if anyone close to me is scheduled to die, can you reschedule, please? Can you rearrange things? I can't handle anymore suffering. I won't make it through another loss." I was angry, numb, tired, and demoralised all at once.

I was totally battle-weary and utterly depleted in every sense of the word.

It felt as though every time I got back up after being knocked down, I would get sucker punched. Life felt unjust and unfair, but I knew that having a pity party or feeling like a victim was not going to change anything. So I dug deep within and found that feisty and gritty chick who was not going to sit back and take it. My only prayer was that somehow God would make a way for me to avoid chemotherapy. I was stripped down to my very core and didn't think I could survive such a violent physical assault. To be honest, I didn't think I had the strength or stamina to survive the treatments.

Something to Smile About

The year after Steve's passing, I didn't even go on one date. Obviously, I had enough going on and I just wasn't looking. I was taking life one day at a time.

I went to a fundraising dinner that May with my parents. This guy who was a friend of the family sat with us, but I was still dealing with my "stuff" and didn't want to be there. I was totally restless and uncomfortable within. Sure he was attractive, but he was engaged, and I'm not one to flirt with someone who is taken. My mind wasn't there *at all* so I left that night never giving him a second thought.

A couple of months later, I needed to get in touch with him to get a hold of his brother. One thing led to another, and we communicated a little through email. I was oblivious to the fact that his relationship had been turbulent from the start and that, at this point, the wedding had been called off and it was over between them.

Meet Chris

On July 28, 2011, Chris and I went on our first "date." I thought nothing of it because he was on the rebound and I was a widow who apparently had cancer. In my mind, I wasn't prime pickings! I wasn't out to "catch" or impress but looked forward to maybe making a new friend. We enjoyed a Dairy Queen treat sitting at the park while we watched local soccer games. We sat there for hours and talked about everything under the sun. It was easy and comfortable to be with him, and conversation seemed to flow naturally.

We kept hanging out occasionally, and the rest is history! I wasn't expecting him to stick around with the cancer and all, but he kept surprising me and loved me regardless of the potential consequences. Chris wasn't necessarily a spiritual type of guy, but after a few dates he personally encountered God's love and presence for the first time—something religion cannot provide! He has since been on his own intimate journey with God.

The Extraction

On September 16, I had a lumpectomy. They may just as well have removed the whole darn breast since I was so small to begin with. There was nothing left of it anyways! The following year I was in and out of the hospital for tests and treatments. I had four major surgeries in one year. I felt like the minute I recovered from one, BAM I was preparing for the next. A lumpectomy, full hysterectomy, reconstruction, and another surgery in my females down under—roughly all within a one-year span.

In November 2011, I started hormone treatments which made my body and emotions do a complete backflip! I was in menopause overnight! It was awful. Since my cancer was hormone induced, I had to bring hormone production in my body to a complete halt. I was highly irritable, moody, angry, and quite depressed. My oncologist took me off the meds for six weeks while I went through radiation to give me a break. Then we played around with the dosage until we found a "happy" and tolerable dose for me.

I was *supposed* to have chemotherapy. I sat down with my oncologist and my aunt that day since my mom couldn't be there. He was a hilarious English doctor who cracked me up every time I saw him. He told me chemotherapy was mandatory. My heart sank, and I was devastated. *However*, listen to this! He said there were about five doctors in Canada who offered an alternative experiential treatment from Austria. I needed to meet four criterias to qualify, and guess what—I met every single one!

140

At that time, the success rate was around 95% (and has only increased since), compared to North American chemo which was about 98%. The game changer for me was that it did not have *any* of the side effects regular chemo had. I broke down immediately because I remembered my one and *only* prayer.

"Please God, *no* chemo!"

I started weeping and told him about my answered prayer. I was a mess, a very happy mess. I felt so undeserving, yet undone by His extravagant love for me. He heard, He answered, and He still loved me just the same even after the mess I had created for myself in years past.

What were the odds of me landing this one out of five Canadian doctors who offered this treatment!? I had a choice to make that day. Either play it safe and do the mainstream treatment option, *or* take a leap of faith and trust this man knows what he is doing! I asked him to tell me what he would recommend if I were his wife or daughter. He said without hesitation that he would encourage the alternative. I was *sold*! The side effects were a walk in the park compared to regular chemo. I got my injections twice a year for three and a half years.

The radiation took a lot more out of me. Towards the end of the six weeks of radiation, I was extremely weak and fatigued with an undercurrent of sadness. Once the treatments were over and the hormone meds stabilised, I gradually started to feel better. My last injection was in fall 2015.

I am Woman, Hear Me Roar!

I had my tubes tied when Steve and I were married. Strangely though, when I had my hysterectomy I remember feeling a huge loss. It lasted a couple of days, but I grieved the impossibility of ever having kids, as well as the loss of having yet another female part getting ripped out of me.

After wrestling with my femininity all my life, it was with Steve's help that I was able to gradually accept and embrace my womanhood. I started wearing makeup and dressing more femininely. With all the progress I was doing internally, I came to a place in my early thirties where I was proud of being a woman. I celebrated it and enjoyed it fully!

I felt ripped off when my breast was removed, and now my insides were on their way out. All the progress I had made to love myself over the years to just now be taken away from me. I felt betrayed by life. It was an intense but luckily short-lived emotional process.

A couple of days after I grieved the loss, I shook off the dust and was ready to move on. I was still a woman and proud of it, no matter how many body parts I was going to have to do away with. I had a resolve in me to just keep standing and moving forward.

Since this alternative chemo was experiential, I had to fill out a questionnaire every three months as part of the research study. That was unpleasant in itself as I remember getting panic attacks while I completed them. Afterwards, I had to consciously tell my brain to stop thinking and move on to something else. I think it fed the reality and fear of what I was actually battling. The big "c" was the enemy I tried to ignore.

I never entertained the thought that I might die, and rarely pondered the harsh reality that I had cancer. I felt myself dissociating from it to a certain degree as a self-preserving mechanism. I went to my appointments and had my treatments but the minute I was out of the hospital I rarely talked or thought about it. I tried to be positive and just kept living my life as if everything was going to be fine.

My high school coach (back from my eating disorder days) and now a dear friend of mine had also been through the wringer. He lent me a book that really helped me fight the big "c" and it was exactly what I needed to read at the beginning of my journey. The author shared how, according to his research, he found a common denominator that many of his cancer patients shared. Many developed cancer 12-24 months *after* they had experienced a traumatic event.

I fit his statistics perfectly.

He also talked about the critical role that faith, staying positive, and healthy relationships with our doctors all play throughout our journey and recovery. I felt so tired and weak that I didn't have the strength to fight. I just went through the motions, trying to fulfil my assignments and appointments for each day. One day at a time.

I was off work for six months on disability. Being a little depressed and in survival mode, I didn't have much energy for friendships. People would occasionally reach out to me, but I had very little desire to respond and engage. I was alienating myself from the outside world except for my immediate family and closest friends. I didn't want anyone's pity, nor did I want to talk about my illness with just anyone. I held my core circle of friends and family closer than ever, and that was all I needed at the time.

I want to encourage those of you who are battling a life-threatening disease to never give up hope. We don't understand "why" some people get healed and others don't make it, or why some people get sick (usually the healthy ones) while others who abuse their bodies seem to have a clean bill of health. Life in itself is a mystery. But it's not what happens to us that matters, instead, it's how we react and manage ourselves throughout our sufferings.

Suffering with Dignity and Grace

To suffer with our chin up, like a champion, with beauty exuding from our being is possible! I personally know a handful of individuals who have done just that. They fight unthinkable battles with strength, dignity and grace and have gained my utmost admiration and respect. They have been such an inspiration to me and many others. And even when you feel so weak that you question whether or not your light still shines, know that it does. No matter how dimly lit you may be, that may be all the light another pilgrim needs to find their way through their own darkness. Your light can pave the way as a beacon of hope where there seems to be no hope.

I'd like to share some of the most helpful things I did throughout this fight that made a huge difference in *my* journey.

1. **LAUGH**. My parents became two of my best friends, and my mom came with me to most of my appointments. She was a real trooper. We called each other Thelma and Louise since the two of us made the perfect recipe for a gong show! We would rarely go to my appointments without some goofy incident taking place. My mom is a riot, hilarious, and has no problem letting her hair down. I will cherish the memories we made in this season for the rest of my life. I just think of her and my heart smiles. There is no one more loving, giving, and sacrificing with a bigger servant heart than my mom! I don't know what I would have done without her. When I think of my cancer, our time together is the first thing that pops into my mind, *not* the suffering!

2. **STAY HEALTHY.** That included eating even when I wasn't hungry and getting proper sleep. I tried to stick to an exercise

program as well, and even though I am far from being who I was before cancer, I have come to accept my new normal. If I never climb Everest or run a marathon, who cares! I am OK with not being a ripped machine and with the fact that I am ageing prematurely due to the menopause spin cycle my body has had to endure. Up until about a year ago, I was still extremely tired and weak. I would exercise for ten minutes (low-impact, may I add) and I would lay down for ten. I would get back up for ten and lay back down for ten. It was so frustrating. But I stuck with it and kept my routine. At least 20–30 minutes a day. Exercise does wonders for our cognitive, physical, and emotional wellbeing.

3. **ATTITUDE.** I stayed positive and kept thinking happy thoughts. I honestly don't think I was in denial or avoidance, rather, it was my way of keeping my head above water. With all the hormonal changes going on, I had no choice but to keep my thoughts and emotions in check. I did my best to love my body throughout all its many changes, scars, and limitations. I had to let go of control and give myself room to make mistakes and be vulnerable. I learned that it was OK to need help from others and to be grateful for everything I had. For me to go down was not an option. However, I felt so weak that I think God was fighting this battle for me, and I just kept showing up with a winning attitude.

4. **MY FAITH.** During this time, my relationship with God was restored. I explored a lot of past hurts and disappointments from the years gone by with the help of my best friend and my current psychotherapist whom I love! I had a very hard time trusting life and trusting God again for *good* to come my way. Whenever I was given a blessing (regardless of its form), I became fearful that it would be taken away from me. I was always expecting the ball to drop. But God in His

loving and gentle approach knew exactly what I needed and gradually restored me to Himself.

5. **DOCTORS.** No one is perfect, and I get that. But I cannot express how much I appreciated each and every single doctor who was put in my path. From my family doctor who went the extra mile with my check-up and potentially saved my life, to my surgeons and oncologists who were all outstanding in care, compassion, and expertise—I am forever grateful for having such quality people in my corner. I never once felt like a number; they always made me feel like I was their only patient in the world. I put my life into their hands knowing God was working through each one. I'm sure it's not a glamorous job and that it can be quite thankless at times. I want to thank each and every one of you for being you and for your exceptional care. Perhaps I am here today writing this book, in part, thanks to you!

Life is good. Life is beautiful. Life is a gift. It is not how we start the race that matters but let's aim to finish the race with dignity and grace. No matter what storm comes our way, we must always remember these words by Victor Hugo:

"Even the darkest night will end and the sun
will rise again."

CHAPTER 11

Turning the Page: A Second Chance at Love and Life

"There are far better things ahead than any
we leave behind."
—C.S. Lewis

We have now arrived at my present chapter, the one that is being lived as we speak. When I look back at the life I've had, I could never have orchestrated any of it or foreseen what was to come. None of us knows what our future holds, but one thing I do know is that no storm or trial lasts forever. I guess I expected that life could be good but never great. You could say that my last couple of years have almost felt like a dream, above and beyond anything I could have asked or imagined!

To this day I still wrestle with the thought that something bad is lurking around the corner or for the next sucker punch to hit. I feel as though life is too good to be true. I fear that if I embrace my present reality it will hurt more when it is lost. But I am gaining faith and strength as I fight off those fears. We are all in process, right?

As much as I loved living in the mountains, I discovered along the way that without love nothing on earth is ever complete or ever feels right. I never accumulated material things, because I preferred to spend my money on adventures and people rather than things.

My whole life I felt like an alien here on earth. I never felt at home anywhere, rather like I didn't belong or there was something missing. I really disliked my hometown and felt like I didn't fit in (which was one of the reasons I never planned on moving back permanently).

All of this changed when I moved back home in 2010. As much as I wanted to return to the mountains during that first year, it just didn't feel like the right thing to do. So I stuck around and waited for clear direction. But that July everything changed when I was diagnosed with cancer and Chris came into the picture. With all the treatments and appointments, I wasn't about to move away. Plus, the more I got to know Chris the fonder I became of this man!

I was drawn to his maturity, stability, and gentleness. He was a blond-haired, blue-eyed stud who loved the outdoors and whose greatest passion in life was hunting. He was a hard-working, loyal and old-fashioned kind of guy. We were both looking for a stable relationship that was drama *free*! The first sign of any mental instability or red flags and I would have been outta there! But that never came, and our friendship naturally progressed into what is now: a beautiful, stable, and loving affair. He is an honest man of integrity, an excellent provider and loving father.

Last year I joined the hunting circus because I figured—if I can't beat 'em, I may as well join 'em! And I love it! My first hunt was a bear hunt (Go big or go home, right?). Chris caught a beauty, but I didn't see anything. Next year I will have my own meat in the freezer for some finger lickin' good bear stew! For those of you who oppose hunting, you can rest in knowing that we don't waste an ounce of our catch.

Although I never wanted kids, when I had my hysterectomy I remember thinking that, if it were possible, I would have considered having a child with Chris because he is such an exceptional father.

His 12-year-old boy Tyler is the son I never had. We call each other "babe," and he is my little man. He is a brilliant, highly sensitive, and gentle boy who will probably make a great hockey commentator one day! He is goofy and so innocent and pure it is refreshing to see.

A Holy Hoedown

The summer of 2014, Chris and I tied the knot. We called it our Holy Hoedown! It was a Western style wedding under the apple trees on my parent's farm. It was magical and could have been a scene out of a movie! I even rode down the "aisle" on my horse with the *Last of the Mohicans* soundtrack playing in the background! I know I am biased because it was our day, but it felt really special, and we know God was there. It was a small and intimate celebration with our family and closest friends. We had homemade pies that our moms and aunts baked and we ended the evening with a hayride through Dad's fields.

Outta Left Field

A few months later, the following fall, I had a curveball thrown at me when my employer wanted us to move across the country so that I could work out of headquarters. With Tyler's mom living in Montreal and Chris working out of Montreal, it was impossible to uproot and split this family.

We could not rip Tyler away from his mom, nor were we going to leave him behind and start over. We didn't have a choice but to decline the offer.

I never realised how difficult it would be to lose a job. I always figured I would just get another one, but that wasn't the case. I had invested so much energy, heart, and passion into this ministry that it felt like a calling more than a job. It was an outlet that allowed me to love and serve others, and I made some incredible friendships there over the years.

I had this lingering sadness and a deep sense of loss that lasted about three months. Until one day in prayer, I felt the release happen, and I was able to let go and move on from that moment. I have to admit that I wasn't quite as passionate as I had once been about my role and was probably more ready for a change than I cared to admit. I believe I was staying for the comfort and safety that the paycheque provided over knowing if that was where I was still meant to be.

For the first time in my life, I was jobless. I didn't know where to go or what to do. I waited for direction and really felt like my next mission was right here inside of me. That is when I decided to pursue my own business as a speaker, mentor, and now author! I've never been happier.

It is only thanks to Chris' stability and provision that I have been able to take this leap of faith. I have never been so stretched in my entire life! Starting a small business is something I never dreamed of doing since I am *not* an entrepreneur at heart.

We don't realise the potential that lays dormant within us until we are forced to tap into it!

I feel as though I am "fledging" (a term used when baby eagles take their first flight away from the nest). I never thought I could fly, but after stepping off this cliff, I am now airborne and exploring uncharted and slightly overwhelming territory. It is both exhilarating and frightening at the same time.

My message and heart is to equip, inspire, and educate individuals on how to build hope and resilience in the face of adversity. Brennan Manning's words ring so true to me:

"If we conceal our wounds out of fear and shame, our inner darkness can neither be illuminated nor become a light for others."

I hope that my story will inspire individuals to make a difference in their own lives but also in those around them. Unfortunately, life doesn't always play fair. None of us has all the answers to our "why" questions. Life happens, and we often feel betrayed and ripped off. Unless we learn to roll with the punches, we will become bitter and be held hostage at our own pity party. We will infest our world with negativity and cynicism.

Never once in my journey have I felt like a victim or asked, "Why me?" When I think of it, why *not* me? What makes me so special that I would be spared any of life's painful struggles? This type of thinking is dangerous because we become victims and self-absorbed navel-gazers. These individuals do not attract sympathy but repel everyone around them.

A friend once asked me why God was making all these bad situations happen to me. I replied that, first of all, none of us have all the answers, but I don't believe God is the source of any evil. He has no sickness in Heaven to give and is not sitting there trying to figure out how to make our lives miserable. He is much better than we think. My personal belief is that there is a war going on between good and evil, and just because we do not see it with our natural eye, doesn't mean it isn't real.

Yes, I went through some challenges, but I know for a fact God was there with me through every single one. I drew my strength from His presence. I knew deep within that He would never leave me nor forsake me, and nothing in all of creation could ever separate me from His love. I wouldn't be here today to tell my tale unless He was alive and kickin' in me!

My Refuge

For the first time in my life, I feel *at home*. And what a heartwarming and comforting feeling that is! I feel settled inside, and I have never known such inner peace. I love our humble little log house in the country with our dog, our horse, and barn cats. We like to call it our funny farm. We have a pond in the backyard where I take our dog for a swim and where probably half of this book was written. My horse has been an incredible source of comfort and quite the shoulder to cry on throughout the years.

Archery, quadding, target shooting, and skidooing are all activities Chris and I enjoy together. We both love anything and everything to do with First Nations people. Our house looks like it's out of an old Western. Chris is the cowboy, and I am the Indian!

Life is simple, peaceful, and beautiful. I cannot begin to express my gratitude to God for everything He has done in my life. From the big and obvious miracles to meeting the quiet desires of my heart, I am simply undone by His undeniable goodness.

He set me free from suicide and depression. He set me free from the trauma with Ben and both eating disorders. He has forgiven me and given me the ability to forgive those who hurt me. He has restored broken relationships and given me new ones that I love and cherish. My relationship with my parents is one I deeply cherish and never take for granted. I thank Him daily for my husband and my little babe, and for this safe haven and refuge I now call home.

Nothing about God or anything He does is mediocre. He makes beauty for ashes and turns our sorrow into joy. He makes all things new and can turn the mess of any storm into a glorious landscape.

Today my heart is finally at rest and my striving has ceased. I am full of joy and I now know peace. Even though I am broken, my spirit is whole. Throughout my lifetime, I recklessly and desperately searched for love in all the wrong places, but I finally found what I was looking for.

I am loved and so are you!

CHAPTER 12

Keeping it Real: From My Heart to Yours

"It's your decisions and not your conditions that
determine your destiny."
—Anthony Robbins

I have not arrived nor do I have all the answers. Like the rest of us, I am a work in progress. I can only continue to be brave enough to express my true self and in turn enable others to do the same. As I continue on my journey, I must continue to offer myself patience and grace to make mistakes and love myself fully in the process.

I hope you will do the same.

We are all in this together. We are all human beings: highly resilient yet deeply fragile individuals. Therefore, we must grow in love, compassion, and grace for one another, because without each other none of us would survive. I get that life can be unfair and just plain suck sometimes. But remember, no one can take away our freedom to choose our attitude in the midst of our suffering. If there was a key to lock you *in* your prison cell, there is a key to let you *out.*

If there was a way *into* your mess, there is a *way out.*
And if I made it through my storms, *so can you.*

The sun may just be hiding behind a cloud, but once that cloud passes, the sun will light the way once again. If you have experienced loss, know that your lost loved one wants nothing but the best for you. Today give yourself permission to move on, to live again, to laugh again, and to love again. Forgive yourself and others and let go of regret. Do not take anyone in your life for granted. You are not going crazy! Healing takes time and there is no predictable timetable for grieving. Be patient with yourself. Live every moment to its fullest as an opportunity to extend love and kindness to the world around you.

> "Every life has a measure of sorrow, and sometimes
> that is what awakens us."
> —Steven Tyler

If you struggle loving yourself, know that you were fearfully and wonderfully made, and there is no flaw in you. I hope you can feel God smiling over you when you read the lyrics from Delirious' song: "God didn't screw up when He made you, He's a father who loves to parade you." Your beauty runs much deeper than your skin. If you feel like an outcast or misfit, *good*! Embrace and celebrate the things that make you unique! It's all about our mindset, so from now on, know that it is OK to be different or weird because last time I checked, most world changers were anything but status quo. The only surgery you need is a heart surgery for the assaults you've endured. You are the only "you" who has ever been or ever will be. Be yourself and stop wasting your energy trying to fill someone else's shoes. There is nothing wrong with you and you do not lack in any way.

> "You have *no rival*."
> —Lisa Bevere

If you are in an abusive relationship, I encourage you to consider your true worth. Every human being deserves to be treated with honour, love, and respect and that includes *you*! If your mate is unable to give you those things because of their own pain, it is not your job to save him or her and put up with their crap. You deserve to be free and live the life you have only dreamed about. It is never too late to make the right decision for you! God is on your side, and you have nothing to fear. If you feel alone, I guarantee there are others around you to care for you and be there for you. Find friends and professionals who will help you establish an exit plan should that be an option. Make sure you do not attempt to leave on your own. Be brave enough to put yourself first and realise you deserve to be cherished. Remember these words by Nelson Mandela,

> "Courage is not the absence of fear
> but the triumph over it."

If you are struggling with any addiction, know that it is just a Band-Aid, and the wound will continue to fester and grow until you get it looked at. When we suffer a physical injury, we see a doctor and get proper care, however, when we suffer an emotional wound, we often do nothing. In turn, we develop coping mechanisms to deal with the discomfort of our soul. I cannot encourage you enough to get help from a friend or a professional. The longer it stays in the dark, the harder it is to conquer the shame that is keeping you silent. It won't get better until you bring it into the light. Life is too short, and if you want it bad enough and keep pursuing your freedom, you will find it. This doesn't have to be your narrative; *you* have the ability to make the right choices today. Will you take the first step? Today could be the first day of the rest of your life! The easy solutions to life's pain and messiness are often the most dangerous. In order to maintain your freedom you will have to stay on the road less traveled. As I mentioned earlier, isolation is an incubator for addictions.

You can either face your pain with courage or hide in the false comfort of your addiction.

Parents, whatever you do, keep the lines of communication open. It may save your family and even save a life. Even when we don't understand our kids or what they are going through, we need to embrace them where they are at and accept their reality as their legitimate personal experience. Sometimes, we need to be vulnerable enough to share our struggles to give others permission to do the same. It's not rocket science. Ask them how they are doing and seek answers that go beyond the surface. If they disclose an issue or struggle, *do not* overreact or belittle their experience. Love them. Be quiet and just listen. Be a safe place for them to land. If it's not you, it will be anyone or anything but you! You may need to learn to "handle the truth"!

For couples, the same idea applies. The more we keep sweeping things under the rug, the more bitter and resentful we become. That results in couples either blowing up at one another or acting out in some form. Even though divorce may be the only option for some, perhaps many marriages could be saved if we attempted to fix what was broken instead of attempting to replace it.

"Be brave enough to start a conversation that *matters*."
—Margaret Wheatly

If you struggle with depression or suicidal thoughts today, please find someone to talk to immediately. Perhaps you are surrounded by people but still feel a sense of emptiness. Or maybe you live alone with a life void of meaningful relationships. Regardless, loneliness, anxiety and depression are rampant in our society today, and there is a way out, but you have to take the first step. You are not a victim so stop feeling sorry for yourself and call off the pity party because *you*, my friend, are awesome! You are the only *you* in this whole world! You deserve to live an abundant and prosperous life full of peace and laughter. You have gifts and a purpose that you alone can fulfil. You are worth the fight, and you add tremendous value to this world. We need you, so don't rob us of the gift that is you! Get out there and figure out your purpose and go be your bodacious self! I know you are hurting deeply and you want to stop the pain but suicide is permanent. Pain is *not*. When we hurt, we become self-absorbed and we feel alone in our relentless torment. I am here to tell you that you are NOT alone.

"If you are looking for a sign not to kill yourself, *this is it*."
—Unknown

I did not overcome any of my struggles because I was special. On the contrary, I am just like everyone else, but I was tenacious for my freedom and refused to let my pain conquer me. The advice I shared were lessons learned from my own fight for survival and hopefully you were able to extract one truth that resonated with you. I wrote this book to encourage you to be brave enough to be vulnerable and to let your *perfectly flawed* self be seen.

Don't let sorrow rob your joy and don't let stress hijack your peace. When we look around, we quickly realise that we all have our own cross to carry. We don't always pick our battles, but we decide whether or not we will let them conquer us. We must limit our navel gazing as it feeds self-pity which ultimately leads to defeat and alienation. We need to keep our perspective in check and continually love and serve our neighbour, because in the end we are all in this together.

You are more powerful than you think, more beautiful than you know, and you are a gift that needs to be opened, and embraced. Do not shrink back and withhold yourself from the world any longer.

May you be filled with hope for today and strength for tomorrow. I pray that you would come to know through experience for yourself the love of God. There is no pit too deep that God's love cannot reach. The Champion of Heaven is on your side, and nothing is impossible for Him.

All of Heaven is cheering you on, and so am I!

Your spouse needs you; your kids need you; the world needs you, so don't you dare give up on us! Your present situation is *not* your permanent destination. Keep moving forward and never ever give up hope. I think it is high time we all give each other permission to be real and vulnerable and grow in compassion and love for one another. By doing so, I believe the world will find safety, grace, healing, and redemption.

You are a masterpiece. You are loved.

From this day forward,
I dare you to be
YOU.

I dare you to be
RAW.

CONCLUSION

"Be yourself; everyone else is already taken."

—Oscar Wilde

NOTES

Chapter 1: All the Ingredients for a Happy Life: What Went Wrong?

1. Lisa Bevere, Without Rival. Grand Rapids, MI: Revell Books, a division of Baker Publishing Group. 2016

Chapter 2: Masked: The Cost of Being an Imposter

1. John Elderedge & Brent Curtis, The Sacred Romance. Nashville, TN: Thomas Nelson Publishers. 1997

Chapter 4: Domestic Violence: Welcome to Hell

1. John Elderedge, Waking the Dead. Nashville, TN: Thomas Nelson Publishers. 2003

Chapter 6: A Fresh Start: Learning to Fly with Broken Wings

1. John Elderedge & Brent Curtis, The Sacred Romance. Nashville, TN: Thomas Nelson Publishers. 1997

Chapter 9: The Collapse: My Road to Recovery

1. John Elderedge, The Journey of Desire. Nashville, TN: Thomas Nelson Publishers. 2000

Chapter 11: Turning the Page: A Second Chance at Love and Life

1. Brennan Manning, Abbas' Child: The Cry of the Heart for Intimate Belonging. Colorado Springs, CO: NavPress. 1994

ACKNOWLEDGEMENTS

Jesus. You have ravished my heart. My wildest and most beautiful adventure has been knowing You.

Kary Oberbrunner. Coach extraordinaire! Without your expertise and guidance this book would have *never* materialized. You're the best! www.karyoberbrunner.com

Chris from JETLAUNCH – You are one in a million. Thank you for your outstanding support, exceptional service and care. www.jetlaunch.net

Abigail. Thank you for your edits. I appreciate you! www.stresslessedits.com

Mila. Thank you for my cover design and for going above the call of duty. www.milagraphicartist.com

Ken & Kelly. Thank you for your honest input, encouragement, edits and support along the way.

Marie-Josée. My photographer and partner in crime. So grateful for your time, ideas, countless edits and much needed laughs throughout this journey. You are a gift.

Danell. My twisted sister! I love you to the moon and back! Thank you for your counsel, wisdom, rebukes, and most of all for your friendship. Thanks for always speaking truth, and helping me tread through the deep waters of my soul. www.oilinc.ca

Monica & Ernie. Thank you for your continued love and support over the years.

Mom & Dad. For being the truest manifestation of love on this side of heaven. I love, honour and appreciate you more than you know.

Chris. Thanks for believing in me and helping me make this book a reality. Without you, none of this would have *ever* been possible. Life with you is a dream come true.

♡melanie willard

Equip. Inspire. Educate.

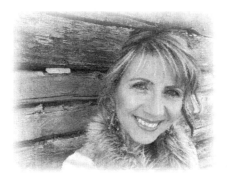

**Bring *Melanie* into
your business or organization**

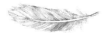

Melanie is an inspirational speaker, author and mentor who helps individuals and organizations grow in resilience and hope in the face of adversity while motivating them to make a difference in their own life and in those around them. She has spoken to thousands of individuals over the last 15 years and has provided one-on-one care to countless individuals going through crisis. Melanie is a top choice for many organizations as she customizes each message to achieve and exceed the objectives and needs of her clients.

Adventurous, passionate, and a fighter who is no stranger to pain, Melanie has overcome many life threatening battles such as cancer, loss, eating disorders, domestic abuse and addictions.

Connect with Melanie at:
melaniewillard.com

Made in the USA
San Bernardino, CA
30 August 2018